Neuromuscular

Rehabilitation Medicine Quick Reference

Ralph M. Buschbacher, MD

Series Editor

Professor, Department of Physical Medicine and Rehabilitation
Indiana University School of Medicine
Indianapolis, Indiana

▣ Spine

Andre N. Panagos

▣ Spinal Cord Injury

Thomas N. Bryce

▣ Traumatic Brain Injury

David X. Cifu and Deborah Caruso

▣ Pediatrics

Maureen R. Nelson

▣ Musculoskeletal, Sports, and Occupational Medicine

William Micheo

▣ Geriatrics

Kevin M. Means and Patrick M. Kortebein

▣ Cancer

Ki Y. Shin

▣ Neuromuscular

Nathan D. Prahlow and John C. Kincaid

Neuromuscular

Rehabilitation Medicine Quick Reference

Editors

Nathan D. Prahlow, MD

Residency Program Director
Assistant Professor of Clinical Physical Medicine and Rehabilitation
Department of Physical Medicine and Rehabilitation
Indiana University School of Medicine
Indianapolis, Indiana

John C. Kincaid, MD

Kenneth L. and Selma G. Earnest Professor of Neurology
Director, Clinical Neurophysiology Fellowship Program
Professor of Physical Medicine and Rehabilitation
Indiana University School of Medicine
Indianapolis, Indiana

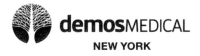

demosMEDICAL

NEW YORK

Visit our website at www.demosmedpub.com

ISBN: 978-1-933864-48-8
e-book ISBN: 978-1-61705-006-0

Acquisitions Editor: Beth Barry
Compositor: Exeter Premedia Services Private Ltd.

Medicine is an ever-changing science. Research and clinical experience are continually expanding our knowledge, in particular our understanding of proper treatment and drug therapy. The authors, editors, and publisher have made every effort to ensure that all information in this book is in accordance with the state of knowledge at the time of production of the book. Nevertheless, the authors, editors, and publisher are not responsible for errors or omissions or for any consequences from application of the information in this book and make no warranty, expressed or implied, with respect to the contents of the publication. Every reader should examine carefully the package inserts accompanying each drug and should carefully check whether the dosage schedules mentioned therein or the contraindications stated by the manufacturer differ from the statements made in this book. Such examination is particularly important with drugs that are either rarely used or have been newly released on the market.

Library of Congress Cataloging-in-Publication Data
Neuromuscular/editors, Nathan Prahlow, John Kincaid.
    p.; cm. — (Rehabilitation medicine quick reference)
  Includes bibliographical references.
  ISBN 978-1-933864-48-8—ISBN 978-1-61705-006-0 (eBook)
 I. Prahlow, Nathan D., editor of compilation.   II. Kincaid, John C., editor of compilation.   III. Series: Rehabilitation medicine quick reference.
  [DNLM: 1. Neuromuscular Diseases—rehabilitation—Handbooks. 2. Movement Disorders—rehabilitation— Handbooks. 3. Neurodegenerative Diseases—rehabilitation—Handbooks. WE 39]
  RC346
  616.8—dc23

                                                  2013034861

Special discounts on bulk quantities of Demos Medical Publishing books are available to corporations, professional associations, pharmaceutical companies, health care organizations, and other qualifying groups.
For details, please contact:

Special Sales Department
Demos Medical Publishing, LLC
11 West 42nd Street, 15th Floor
New York, NY 10036
Phone: 800-532-8663 or 212-683-0072
Fax: 212-941-7842
E-mail: specialsales@demosmedpub.com

Printed in the United States of America by Bradford and Bigelow.
13 14 15 16 17 / 5 4 3 2 1

Contents

II   Polyneuropathies

III   Neuromuscular Junction

IV   Radiculopathies/Plexopathies

V   Motor Neuron Diseases

VI   Muscle Diseases

VII   Movement Disorders

Series Foreword

The Rehabilitation Medicine Quick Reference (RMQR) series is dedicated to the busy clinician. While we all strive to keep up with the latest medical knowledge, there are many times when things come up in our daily practices that we need to look up. Even more important . . . look up quickly.

Those aren't the times to do a complete literature search, or to read a detailed chapter, or review an article. We just need to get a quick grasp of a topic that we may not see routinely or just to refresh our memory. Sometimes a subject comes up that is outside our usual scope of practice, but that may still impact our care. It is for such moments that this series has been created.

Whether you need to quickly look up what a Tarlov cyst is, or you need to read about a neurorehabilitation complication or treatment, RMQR has you covered.

RMQR is designed to include the most common problems found in a busy practice and also a lot of the less common ones as well.

I was extremely lucky to have been able to assemble an absolutely fantastic group of editors. They, in turn, have harnessed an excellent set of authors. So what we have in this series is, I hope and believe, a tremendous reference set to be used often in daily clinical practice. As series editor, I have of course been privy to these books before actual publication. I can tell you that I have already started to rely on them in my clinic—often. They have helped me become more efficient in practice.

Each chapter is organized into succinct facts, presented in a bullet point style. The chapters are set up in the same way throughout all of the volumes in the series, so once you get used to the format, it is incredibly easy to look things up.

And while the focus of the RMQR series is, of course, rehabilitation medicine, the clinical applications are much broader.

I hope that each reader grows to appreciate the RMQR series as much as I have. I congratulate a fine group of editors and authors on creating readable and useful texts.

Ralph M. Buschbacher, MD

A broad group of diagnoses is encompassed by the term "Neuromuscular Disease." The frequency with which clinicians encounter these conditions ranges widely, from the common (carpal tunnel syndrome, with an incidence of 1 in 20) to the extremely rare (congenital myasthenic syndrome). The severity of the illnesses similarly varies dramatically, from generally benign (hereditary neuropathy with liability to pressure palsies), to universally fatal (spinal muscular atrophy, type 1). The pathophysiology of the disease processes includes abnormalities in the central nervous system, neuronal cell bodies, peripheral nerves, neuromuscular junction, and the muscles themselves. Causes may be environmental, inherited, developmental, age related, overuse, injury, or exposure to poisons. Treatment options might include supportive care, medical management of symptoms, therapeutic modalities, immune modulation, injections, surgeries, or alternative medicine practices.

Despite all of the variability one encounters when leafing through this volume in the Rehabilitation Medicine Quick Reference (RMQR) series, one thing is clear: Each of these diagnoses affects the patient's function. Therefore, the treating clinician must have the improvement of function as a primary goal. Although functional improvement is an obvious goal when one has a peripheral nerve injury that has undergone corrective surgery, one must also focus on functional improvement in the patient with a condition that will be lifelong or even fatal: For the patient with amyotrophic lateral sclerosis, functional mobility may be improved when a power wheelchair is utilized.

Although the RMQR series as a whole focuses on the diagnoses encountered in the field of physical medicine and rehabilitation, this volume explores diagnoses often managed by our colleagues in the field of neurology. Just as we have the most excellent arrangement where both the physiatrist and the neurologist may serve as electrodiagnosticians, this volume serves to facilitate the great interaction between these two fields in the treatment of patients with neuromuscular diseases.

Nathan D. Prahlow, MD
John C. Kincaid, MD

Acknowledgments

This project grew from a seemingly innocent question asked by series editor Dr. Ralph Buschbacher: "Would you be interested in helping put together another book on EMG?" For this opportunity and for his assistance in editing and revising, I thank Ralph, and look forward to future collaborations! I also thank my family—Julie, Joshua, Caleb, and Jonathan—for supporting me and giving me the time to work on this project.

Nathan D. Prahlow, MD

I thank Dr. Buschbacher for asking me to author this volume of the series, and Beth Barry for her infinite patience during the editorial process. I appreciate the many great things I have learnt from my colleagues in physical medicine and rehabilitation.

John C. Kincaid, MD

Contributors

Matthew Axtman, DO
Orthopaedics & Sports Medicine
Spectrum Health
Grand Rapids, Michigan

Cynthia L. Bodkin, MD
Assistant Professor of Clinical Neurology
IU School of Medicine
Department of Neurology
Indiana University Health Physicians
Indianapolis, Indiana

Shashank J. Davé, DO, FAAPMR
Clinical Assistant Professor
Department of Physical Medicine and Rehabilitation
Department of Neurology
Co-Chief Physical Medicine and Rehabilitation
Indiana University School of Medicine
Indianapolis, Indiana

Gentry Dodd, MD
Resident Physician
Department of Physical Medicine and Rehabilitation
Indiana University School of Medicine
Indianapolis, Indiana

John C. Kincaid, MD
Kenneth L. and Selma G. Earnest Professor of Neurology
Director, Clinical Neurophysiology Fellowship Program
Professor of Physical Medicine and Rehabilitation
Indiana University School of Medicine
Indianapolis, Indiana

Nathan D. Prahlow, MD
Residency Program Director
Assistant Professor of Clinical Physical Medicine and
    Rehabilitation
Department of Physical Medicine and Rehabilitation
Indiana University School of Medicine
Indianapolis, Indiana

Gabriel Smith, MD
Resident Physician
Department of Physical Medicine and Rehabilitation
Mayo School of Graduate Medical Education
Rochester, Minnesota

Susan X. Yu, DO
Department of Occupational Health Services
Kaiser Permanente
Los Angeles, California

Shangming Zhang, MD, FAAPMR
Assistant Professor
Medical Director, Physical Medicine and Rehabilitation
    Outpatient Clinic
Department of Physical Medicine and Rehabilitation
Penn State Milton S. Hershey Medical Center
Penn State College of Medicine
Hershey, Pennsylvania

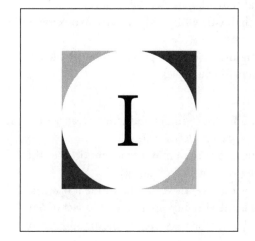

Mononeuropathies

Axillary Neuropathy

John C. Kincaid MD

Description
Syndrome due to a lesion of the axillary nerve

Etiology
- Compression of the nerve in its course posterior and inferior to the shoulder joint, during traumatic shoulder dislocation, occurring in approximately 40% of cases
- Inflammatory neuritis as a component of brachial plexitis
- Compression of the nerve due to positioning in surgery or other instances of prolonged sedation/nonresponsiveness
- Entrapment as the nerve exits the axilla through the quadrilateral space

Epidemiology
Most often occurs as a component of trauma to the shoulder

Pathogenesis
- Demyelination and axonopathy due to the primary pathogenesis
- Inflammatory neuritis

Risk Factors
Traumatic shoulder dislocation

Clinical Features
- Weakness of shoulder abduction
- Atrophy of the deltoid: note that the anterior and medial components of the muscle are supplied by the anterior branch of the nerve, whereas the posterior aspect of the muscle is supplied by the posterior branch of the nerve.
- Sensory loss over the surface of the midportion of the muscle due to the involvement of the anterior branch of the nerve, and over the surface of the posterior aspect of the muscle due to the involvement of the posterior branch.
- Weakness and atrophy of the teres minor due to involvement of the posterior branch of the nerve

Natural History
Slow improvement over months to 2 years if reinnervation is successful

Diagnosis

Differential diagnosis
- Arthritis of the shoulder joint
- Inflammation or degeneration of the tendons/muscles of the shoulder
- Cervical radiculopathy at the C5 level
- Brachial plexitis with predominant involvement of the axillary nerve
- Focal manifestation of a polyneuropathy such as mononeuritis multiplex

History
- Abrupt onset of shoulder abduction weakness in the setting of trauma to the shoulder
- Onset during recurrent, vigorous motions of the shoulder, such as ball pitching
- Onset over a several-week time frame if brachial plexitis is the etiology: spontaneous onset of pain followed several weeks later by motor and sensory deficits
- Surface numbness over the lateral and posterior aspects of the deltoid

Physical examination
- Weakness of arm abduction and atrophy of the deltoid; note that the anterior branch of the nerve supplies the anterior and middle portions of the muscle, whereas the posterior branch supplies the posterior aspect of the muscle.
- Impairment of cutaneous sensation over the lateral and/or posterior aspects of the deltoid
- Mild weakness of external rotation of the shoulder due to teres minor involvement in which the posterior branch of the nerve is affected

Testing
- Needle EMG of the deltoid and adjacent muscles of the shoulder to assess the scope and severity of involvement and to help define prognosis during follow-up
- Nerve conduction study of the axillary nerve if the practitioner is skilled in the technique
- Imaging of the shoulder joint and associated muscles/tendons

Treatment

- Manage lesions of the shoulder joint and associated muscles/tendons, including anti-inflammatory and analgesic medications for pain
- Antineuropathic pain medications usually do not significantly improve the symptoms if the lesion is neurogenic.
- Anti-inflammatory medications may reduce shoulder pain if joint or soft tissue components are the predominant etiology.
- Physical therapy to address range of motion and strengthening

Prognosis

Improvement in motor and sensory deficits over months

Suggested Readings

Stewart, John D. *Focal Peripheral Neuropathies*. 4th ed. (pp. 173–180). West Vancouver, BC, Canada: JBJ Publishing; 2010.

Wilbourn AJ, Ferrante MA. Upper limb neuropathies. In: Dyck PJ, Thomas PK, eds. *Peripheral Neuropathy*. 4th ed. (pp. 1469–1471). Philadelphia, PA: Elsevier; 2005.

Facial Neuropathy (Bell's Palsy)

John C. Kincaid MD

Description
Syndrome due to a focal lesion of the facial nerve

Etiology
- Inflammatory neuritis within the facial canal of the temporal bone: idiopathic or as a manifestation of an immunity altering condition, such as of Lyme disease or sarcoidosis
- Nerve trauma from temporal bone fractures, parotid surgery, mandibular fractures, or repair thereof, acoustic neuroma surgery
- Compression by neoplasms: parotid lesions, invasive lesions of the temporal bone

Epidemiology
Yearly incidence of about 20 cases per 100,000 of population

Pathogenesis
- Autoimmune inflammation of the nerve
- Trauma to neighboring structures such as the mandible, temporal bone
- Compression secondary to infiltration by neoplastic cells from adjacent structures such as the parotid gland or temporal bone

Risk Factors
- Diabetes
- Pregnancy
- Melkersson-Rosenthal syndrome: recurring attacks of facial edema, facial paralysis, and lingua plicata
- Herpes Zoster outbreak involving the sensory innervation of the ear: Ramsay Hunt syndrome

Clinical Features
- A unilateral lesion is more common
- Right- or left-side involvement of equal incidence
- Facial weakness in a "peripheral pattern," that is, upper, mid, and lower facial innervated muscles equally affected

Natural History
Improvement in the majority of patients over a 3-week period after onset.

Diagnosis

Differential diagnosis
Central nervous system lesion of the facial motor pathways: lower face is predominantly involved

History
- Pain in the ear or retroauricular area for hours to a day preceding onset of facial weakness
- Unilateral facial weakness, which tends to be abrupt in onset
- Vague sensory symptoms in the face: "numbness."
- Abnormal taste sensations
- Alerted hearing

Physical examination
- Unilateral weakness of forehead, periorbital, and perioral muscles plus the platysma
- Normal sensation in the trigeminal territory
- Herpetic vesicles in the external ear (rare)

Testing
- Facial nerve conduction studies performed 14 or more days after onset can help define lesions as to predominantly demyelinating versus axonal pathology
- Needle EMG done 21 or more days after the onset can help distinguish demyelinating versus axonal predominance: fibrillation potentials indicate axonal pathology, whereas the preserved ability to activate some voluntary potentials indicates at least some degree of preserved axonal continuity
- Imaging studies if deficits persist beyond 6 months

Treatment
- Oral steroids begun in the first 48 to 72 hours in patients with complete paralysis have a higher chance of recovery
- The addition of an anti-herpes virus agent-like acyclovir does not improve the outcome
- Surgical decompression of the facial canal within the first 14 days of onset does not seem to improve the long-term outcome

Prognosis

- 70+ % have a full recovery
- Up to 10% may have residual weakness and may experience reinnervation phenomena, such as synkinetic movements, abnormal tearing, or hemifacial spasm

Suggested Readings

Klein C. Diseases of the seventh cranial nerve. In Dyck PJ, Thomas PK, eds. *Peripheral Neuropathy*. 4th ed. (pp. 1219-1252). Philadelphia, PA: Elsevier; 2005.

Sullivan F, Swam I, et al. Early treatment with prednisolone or acyclovir in Bell's Palsy. *N Engl J Med* 2007;357:1598–1607.

Femoral Neuropathy

John C. Kincaid MD

Description
Syndrome due to a lesion of the femoral nerve along its course from the level of the psoas muscle into the thigh

Etiology
- Compression by hematoma or other masses along the nerve from the level of the lateral border of the psoas caudally through the level of the inguinal ligament
- Nerve trauma during intra-abdominal surgery, hip arthroplasty, hip fracture, or vascular access procedures in the groin or thigh
- Penetrating injury from gun shots or stab wounds
- Diabetic or idiopathic radiculoplexopathy with predominant involvement of the femoral nerve

Epidemiology
Less common than lesions of the sciatic nerve

Pathogenesis
- External compression of the nerve with resulting demyelination and axonopathy
- Direct trauma during penetrating injury
- Inflammatory neuritis or vasculitis affecting the vasa nervorum

Risk Factors
- Intra-abdominal surgery
- Hip arthroplasty
- Vascular access procedures through the femoral artery or vein

Clinical Features
- Weakness of knee extension
- Hip flexion may also be weak if the rectus femoris is involved
- Paresthesia and sensory loss in anterior thigh and medial lower leg (saphenous nerve distribution)
- Pain of variable intensity in the groin and thigh

Natural History
May improve over many months depending on the nature of the lesion

Diagnosis

Differential diagnosis
- Arthritis involving the hip joint
- Lumbar radiculopathy involving the 2nd, 3rd, or 4th nerve roots
- Lumbar plexopathy with predominant involvement of the femoral nerve

History
- Acute onset when the lesion occurs intraoperatively or due to penetrating trauma
- Onset over hours to a few days when retroperitoneal hematoma formation is the etiology
- Onset over weeks if plexitis is the cause

Physical examination
- Weakness of knee extension
- Mild weakness of knee extension (major weakness of hip flexion suggests a proximal lesion at or proximal to the level of the femoral branch to the iliacus)
- Absence or reduction of the knee muscle stretch reflex
- Atrophy of the quadriceps in long-standing cases
- Loss of sensation in the anterior thigh and medial lower leg
- Loss of sensation also including the lateral thigh suggests a proximal lesion at the level of the psoas where femoral and lateral cutaneous axons are adjacent
- Normal strength in leg adduction and ankle extension

Testing
- Needle EMG shows denervation in the quadriceps but normal results in the hip adductors and tibialis anterior
- Conduction study of the femoral nerve may show reduced amplitude of the compound muscle action potential (CMAP) or absence of the response
- Imaging of the hip joint and pelvis when fractures are suspected
- Imaging of the pelvis to identify hematoma, abscess, or neoplastic lesions along the course of the nerve

Treatment
- Consideration of surgical intervention when retroperitoneal or femoral sheath hematoma is the etiology

- Analgesics if neuropathic pain is a major feature
- Physical therapy to maximize muscle strength improvement
- Knee bracing to compensate for quadriceps weakness

Prognosis

Improvement in sensory and motor symptoms may occur over months

Suggested Readings

Katirji B, Wilbourn A. Mononeuropathies of the lower limb. In: Dyck PJ, Thomas PK, eds. *Peripheral Neuropathy.* 4th ed. (pp. 1487–1510). Philadelphia, PA: Elsevier; 2005

Stewart, John D. *Focal Peripheral Neuropathies.* 4th ed. (pp. 540–555). West Vancouver, BC, Canada: JBJ Publishing; 2010.

Inguinal Neuropathies (Iliohypogastric, Ilioinguinal, and Genitofemoral Nerves)

John C. Kincaid MD

Description

Syndrome due to a focal lesion of these nerves in their course from the psoas to the groin

Etiology

- Trauma during intrapelvic surgery or compression by retroperitoneal masses
- Trauma to or entrapment of the nerve during inguinal herniorrhaphy or other surgical procedures on the lower anterior abdominal wall

Epidemiology

The ilioinguinal nerve may be traumatized in up to 20% of patients undergoing inguinal hernia repair.

Pathogenesis

Local demyelination and axonopathy due to compression of or trauma to the nerve

Risk Factors

- Inguinal herniorrhaphy

Clinical Features

- Pain in lower anterior abdomen and groin
- Numbness and paresthesias in the groin

Natural History

Symptoms tend to be persistent

Diagnosis

Differential diagnosis

- Hip arthritis or bursitis
- Radiculopathy involving the 1st lumbar level
- Upper lumbar plexopathy

History

- Pain in the groin
- Numbness and paresthesia in the lower anterior abdomen, inguinal region, and/or scrotum/labia

Physical examination

- Decreased light touch and pin prick sensation in the:
  - Lateral hip and/or lower anterior abdomen (iliohypogastric)
  - Inguinal canal and upper part of the scrotum or labia (ilioinguinal)
  - Anterior proximal thigh and upper part of the scrotum or labia (genitofemoral)
- Normal strength of hip flexion, leg abduction, and adduction and knee extension
- Normal patellar muscle stretch reflex
- Unilateral impairment or absence of the cremasteric reflex (genitofemoral)

Testing

- Nerve conduction studies of these nerves are not technically reliable
- Needle EMG of proximal leg and upper lumbar paraspinal muscles should be normal
- Imaging studies of the spine and pelvis to investigate the L1 spinal and retroperitoneal region

Treatment

- Analgesic, anti-inflammatory, and antineuropathic pain medications may help
- Re-exploration of the inguinal canal when onset follows inguinal herniorrhaphy

Prognosis

- Inguinal pain often persists long term

Suggested Readings

Amid PK, Hiatt JR. New understanding of the causes and surgical treatment of postherniorrhaphy inguinodynia and orchalgia. *J Am Coll Surg.* 2007;205:381–385.

Stewart, John D. *Focal Peripheral Neuropathies.* 4th ed. (pp. 576–591). West Vancouver, BC, Canada: JBJ Publishing; 2010.

Intercostobrachial Neuropathy

John C. Kincaid MD

Description
Syndrome due to a lesion of the intercostobrachial nerve

Etiology
- Nerve trauma during surgery in the axilla or compression by an invading neuroplasm

Epidemiology
- Chronic postmastectomy pain is felt by 20% to 65% of those undergoing breast surgery for cancer
- An estimated 33% of these cases are due to intercostobrachial neuropathy
- The intercostobrachial nerve is damaged in 80% to 100% of breast cancer surgeries

Pathogenesis
- Nerve trauma during axillary lymph node dissections in breast cancer surgery
- Compression of the nerve by neoplastic infiltration from apical lung tumors

Risk Factors
- Surgical treatment of breast cancer with axillary lymph node dissection

Clinical Features
- Pain in axilla
- Paresthesia and sensory loss in the axilla and proximal medial arm

Natural History
- Onset immediately postoperatively or within a few months of the surgical procedure
- Symptoms tend to be persistent

Diagnosis

Differential diagnosis
- Lesion of the shoulder joint or associated soft tissue
- Radiculopathy involving the T1 or T2 levels

History
- Pain in the axilla perceived as surface or deep
- Numbness and/or paresthesia in the axilla and proximal medial arm
- Swelling of the arm due to disturbance of normal lymph flow

Physical examination
- Decreased sensation to light touch or pin prick in axilla and proximal medial arm
- Strength of shoulder and proximal arm muscles should be normal

Testing
- Nerve conduction studies of median, ulnar, and medial antebrachial cutaneous nerves to evaluate for lower brachial plexopathy
- Needle EMG of C8 and T1 muscles to evaluate for lower brachial plexopathy or lower cervical radiculopathy

Treatment
- Analgesic, anti-inflammatory, and antineuropathic pain medications in an attempt to lessen neuropathic pain
- Nerve block of the intercostobrachial nerve to verify neurogenic causation and to localize the lesion
- Physical therapy to optimize shoulder motions

Prognosis
- Symptoms tend to be persistent

Suggested Readings
Stewart, John D. *Focal Peripheral Neuropathies*. 4th ed. (pp. 183–185). West Vancouver, BC, Canada: JBJ Publishing; 2010.

Torresan RZ, Cabello C, et al. Impact of preservation of the intercostobrachial nerve in axillary lymphadenopathy due to breast cancer. *Breast J.* 2003; 9:398–392.

Lateral Femoral Cutaneous Neuropathy (Meralgia Paresthetica)

John C. Kincaid MD

Description

Syndrome due to a focal lesion of the lateral cutaneous nerve of the thigh

Etiology

- Compression within the pelvis by retroperitoneal mass, hematoma, or surgical retractors
- Trauma at the level of the inguinal ligament by surgical procedures or compression of the nerve by lithotomy positioning, tight clothing, obesity, bulky objects in front pants pockets, or prolonged/recurrent leaning against external structures at the height of the groin or upper thigh
- Idiopathic (most common)

Epidemiology

Likely the most common lower extremity mononeuropathy

Pathogenesis

Local demyelination and in more severe lesions axonopathy due to external compression of the nerve

Risk Factors

- Obesity
- Intra-pelvic or inguinal surgery
- Wearing overly tight pants

Clinical Features

- Burning and numb-type paresthesias in the lateral thigh
- Loss of sensation in the lateral thigh

Natural History

May improve over months with weight reduction

Diagnosis

Differential diagnosis

- Arthritis involving the hip joint
- Trochanteric bursitis
- Lumbar radiculopathy at the L1 or L2 level
- Lumbar plexopathy
- Femoral neuropathy

History

- Symptoms are more often unilateral
- Abrupt onset of lateral thigh pain and numbness following intra-pelvic or inguinal surgery
- Gradual onset when associated with obesity, wearing overly tight pants or in idiopathic cases
- Cutaneous hypersensitivity in the lateral thigh
- Normal strength in hip and thigh functions

Physical examination

- Decreased sensation to light touch or pin prick in lateral thigh
- Normal strength in hip flexion, knee extension, and leg adduction
- Normal bulk of quadriceps
- Normal knee muscle stretch reflex
- Pressure at the level of the inguinal ligament at or just medial to the anterior superior iliac spine may reproduce or worsen the lateral thigh paresthesia
- No pain with palpation of the greater trochanter

Testing

- Nerve conduction studies of the lateral cutaneous nerve are technically reliable only in thin individuals and a normal response must be present on the contralateral side for the values of the symptomatic side to be interpretable
- Nerve conduction studies in normomorphic or heavy individuals are not reliable
- The expected abnormality in conduction studies is reduction of the nerve action potential amplitude or absence of a measureable response
- Needle EMG of the quadriceps and adductor muscles should be normal
- Imaging study of the pelvis if a retroperitoneal lesion is a possible cause

Treatment

- Analgesic, anti-inflammatory, and antineuropathic pain medications usually do not significantly improve the symptoms
- Manage intra-pelvic lesions, which may be compressing the nerve
- Weight reduction
- Local anesthetic block of the nerve for diagnostic and potentially therapeutic purposes
- Surgical decompression of the nerve at the inguinal ligament

Prognosis

Improvement over months if an identifiable lesion is present and management such as weight loss, therapeutic nerve block, or surgical decompression can be instituted

Suggested Readings

Stewart, John D. *Focal Peripheral Neuropathies*. 4th ed. (pp. 556–567). West Vancouver, BC, Canada; 2010.

Wiezer M, Franssen H, et al. Meralgia paresthetica: Differential diagnosis and follow-up. *Muscle Nerve.* 1996;19:522–524.

Long Thoracic Neuropathy

John C. Kincaid MD

Description
Syndrome due to a lesion of the long thoracic nerve

Etiology
- Trauma to the nerve as a component of injury to the shoulder and surrounding soft tissues
- Inflammatory neuritis as component of brachial plexitis
- Idiopathic

Epidemiology
Uncommon but classic lesion

Pathogenesis
- Demyelination and axonopathy due to primary etiology
- Inflammatory neuritis
- Traction injury to the nerve

Risk Factors
- Other trauma to the shoulder region
- Wearing heavy backpack

Clinical Features
- Weakness of flexion or abduction motions of the shoulder
- Acute pain in the shoulder or arm preceding the onset of muscular dysfunction
- Long-term pain in the shoulder and proximal arm during shoulder motions

Natural History
- Pain and muscular dysfunction may improve over months to about 1 year

Diagnosis
Differential diagnosis
- Arthritis of the shoulder
- Rotator cuff syndrome due to inflammation or degeneration of the tendons of the parascapular muscles
- Acute brachial plexopathy/plexitis
- Spinal accessory neuropathy

History
- Pain in the arm/proximal shoulder area
- Weakness of flexion and abduction motions of the shoulder (due to poor stabilization of the scapula)

Physical examination
- Winging of the medial border of the scapula during flexion and protraction motions of the shoulder
- Mild diffuse weakness in flexion and protraction motions of the shoulder
- The bulk and strength of other parascapular muscles should be normal if the lesion is limited to the long thoracic nerve.
- Cutaneous sensation in the shoulder and arm areas should be normal if the lesion is limited to the long thoracic nerve.

Testing
- Needle EMG of the serratus anterior as well as parascapular and proximal arm muscles
- Nerve conduction study of the long thoracic nerve if the practitioner is experienced with the technique

Treatment
- Analgesic and anti-inflammatory medications may improve the shoulder/proximal arm pain
- Orthopedic or physical medicine evaluation of the shoulder to rule out a lesion of the joint or rotator cuff
- Imaging of the shoulder to rule out a lesion of the shoulder joint or rotator cuff
- Physical therapy to optimize strength of other parascapular muscles
- Muscle transfer surgery if severe weakness and associated shoulder motion dysfunction persist beyond about 6 months

Prognosis
- Improvement of shoulder motion and reduction of pain may occur over months to about 1 year

Suggested Readings
Friedenberg SM, Zimprich T. The natural history of long thoracic and spinal accessory neuropathies. *Muscle Nerve*. 2002;25:535–539.
Stewart, John D. *Focal Peripheral Neuropathies*. 4th ed. (pp. 162–167). West Vancouver, BC, Canada: JBJ Publishing; 2010.

Medial Antebrachial Cutaneous Neuropathy

John C. Kincaid MD

Description
Syndrome due to a lesion of the medial cutaneous nerve of the forearm

Etiology
- Penetrating injury in the upper arm
- Trauma to the nerve during surgery on the ulnar nerve at the elbow
- Compression in the lower brachial plexus of the fascicles, which will give rise to the medial cutaneous nerve

Epidemiology
Rare lesion: encountered most often as a complication of surgery for ulnar neuropathy at the elbow

Pathogenesis
Direct trauma to the nerve during penetrating injuries or surgery on the ulnar nerve at the elbow with resulting demyelination and axonal damage

Risk Factors
Surgery for ulnar neuropathy at the elbow

Clinical Features
- Pain in the medial elbow, which may be provocable by elbow motion or palpation of or pressure on the entrapment site
- Tingling and/or numb-type paresthesias in the medial forearm extending from the elbow to the wrist
- Sensory and motor functions of the ulnar nerve should be normal

Natural History
- May improve over several months

Diagnosis

Differential diagnosis
- Medial epicondylitis
- Degenerative arthritis of the elbow
- Cervical radiculopathy involving the C8 or T1 nerve roots
- Lower trunk or medial cord brachial plexopathy
- Neurogenic thoracic outlet syndrome
- Ulnar neuropathy elbow
- Focal manifestation of polyneuropathy

History
- Onset following penetrating injury of the arm or following surgery to treat ulnar neuropathy at the elbow
- Pain in the medial elbow region and along the surgical scar line if the lesion arises postoperatively

Physical examination
- Decreased sensation to light touch or pin prick in medial forearm
- Normal sensation in the ulnar territories of the hand and digits unless an ulnar lesion preceded the onset of the medial cutaneous nerve lesion
- Normal muscle bulk and strength in ulnar and median hand intrinsic muscles unless deficits are attributable to a prior ulnar neuropathy
- Absence of exam features of Horner's syndrome
- Tinel's sign and pain provocable by palpation may be present at the site of nerve entrapment/injury

Testing
- Local anesthetic block of the nerve confirms the origin of the pain and paresthesias
- Ulnar and median conduction studies should be normal unless a lesion of either of those nerves preceded onset of the medial cutaneous neuropathy
- Needle EMG of C8–T1 supplied ulnar, median, and distal radial muscles should be normal unless a lesion of those nerves was present prior to the onset of the medial cutaneous neuropathy
- Imaging of the cervical spine and brachial plexus by magnetic resonance imaging (MRI) should be normal as should cervical spine films done to identify cervical ribs

Treatment
- Antineuropathic pain medications
- Therapeutic nerve block

- Occupational therapy for desensitization
- Exploration of the nerve at the site of injury for release of entrapment or resection of a neuroma if pain and hypersensitivity persist beyond 6 months

Prognosis

- Improvement over several months with conservative treatments such as massage and desensitization

- Improvement in pain and allodynia if surgery is performed for patients not responding to conservative management

Suggested Readings

Dellon A, Mackinnon S. Injury to the medial antebrachial cutaneous nerve during cubital tunnel surgery. *J Hand Surg (Br)*. 1985;10:33–36.

Stewart, John D. *Focal Peripheral Neuropathies*. 4th ed. (pp. 183–193).West Vancouver, BC, Canada: JBJ Publishing; 2010.

Median Neuropathy—Anterior Interosseous Neuropathy (Kiloh-Nevin Syndrome)

John C. Kincaid MD

Description

Syndrome due to a lesion of the anterior interosseous branch of the median nerve

Etiology

- Inflammation of the anterior interosseous nerve or the fascicles within the main trunk of the median nerve, which will give rise to the anterior interosseous nerve
- Entrapment/compression of the anterior interosseous branch of the median nerve by fibrous band components of forearm muscles such as the pronator teres or flexor digitorum superficialis
- Penetrating trauma, which selectively or predominantly involves this branch of the median nerve

Epidemiology

Rare lesion, encounter about once annually in an 1800-patient per year EMG laboratory.

Pathogenesis

- Demyelination and axonopathy of the fascicles within the main trunk of the median nerve or the brachial plexus, which give rise to the anterior interosseous branch

Risk Factors

None

Clinical Features

- Weakness in flexion of the tip of the thumb and index finger
- Pain in the forearm or upper arm
- No sensory deficits

Natural History

- May improve over months if reinnervation is successful

Diagnosis

Differential diagnosis

- Proximal median neuropathy predominantly involving the anterior interosseous fascicles
- Cervical radiculopathy involving the 6th or 7th nerve roots
- Upper or middle trunk brachial plexopathy
- Local manifestation of a polyneuropathy such as mononeuritis multiplex or multifocal motor neuropathy
- Rupture or laceration of the tendon of the flexor pollicis longus

History

- Weakness of flexion of the tip of the thumb and index finger producing inability to properly form an "OK" gesture
- Pain in the forearm, elbow, upper arm, or shoulder preceding onset of muscle weakness by days to a few weeks in case of autoimmune inflammatory neuritis
- No sensory symptoms such as numbness or tingling in the median sensory areas

Physical examination

- Weakness of flexion of the tip of the thumb, index, and at times middle finger
- Normal strength in median innervated hand intrinsic muscles: abductor pollicis brevis, opponens pollicis, and the first two lumbricals
- Normal strength in median innervated forearm muscles such as pronator teres and flexor carpi radialis
- Normal sensation in the median nerve and C6 or C7 territories

Testing

- Standard median motor and sensory nerve conduction studies should be normal
- Needle EMG should show denervation in forearm muscles supplied by the anterior interosseous branch of the median nerve and normal results in hand and forearm muscles supplied by the main trunk of the nerve
- Conduction studies can be performed in the anterior interosseous branch if the practitioner is skilled/confident in the technique: the expected findings would be reduction of the compound muscle action potential (CMAP) from the flexor pollicis longus and perhaps prolongation of the latency from the stimulus site to the muscle.

- Imaging studies of the distal humerus to rule out a supracondylar bone spur
- Magnetic resonance imaging (MRI) of the cervical spine to rule out radiculopathy at the C6 or C7 level

Treatment
- Reduce repetitive elbow/forearm activity such as repetitive pronation/supination
- Conservative observation over 3 to 6 months while watching for recovery in spontaneous onset cases
- Repeat needle EMG at 8 to 12 weeks after onset can reveal whether reinnervation is occurring

- Surgical exploration of the elbow/proximal forearm if no clinical or EMG signs of beginning recovery are present by 3 to 6 months after onset

Prognosis
- Improvement over months to about 2 years in spontaneous onset cases

Suggested Readings
Stevens JC. Median neuropathy. In: Dyck PJ, Thomas PK, eds. *Peripheral Neuropathy*. 4th ed. (pp. 1453–1454). Philadelphia, PA: Elsevier; 2005.

Stewart, John D. *Focal Peripheral Neuropathies*. 4th ed. (pp. 207–214). West Vancouver, BC Canada: JBJ Publishing; 2010.

Median Neuropathy—In the Arm to Mid-Forearm

John C. Kincaid MD

Description

Focal lesion of the median nerve at sites proximal to the level of the carpal tunnel

Etiology

- Penetrating injuries during venous or arterial access procedures in the antecubital fossa
- Compression injury due to fractures of the distal humerus or proximal radius
- Entrapment by aberrant bony spicules arising from the distal medial humerus (the supracondylar spur) or by muscular and fascial structures just distal to the elbow (pronator syndrome)

Epidemiology

Very rare lesion

Pathogenesis

Demyelination and axonopathy due to compression, penetration, or vascular compromise

Risk Factors

- Venipuncture or arterial puncture in the antecubital fossa
- Fractures of the humerus or elbow
- Vascular access creation in the forearm for dialysis

Clinical Features

- Weakness in the median nerve hand functions: thumb abduction and opposition, flexion of the metacarpophalangeal (MCP) joint of digits II and III
- Weakness of forearm pronation, wrist flexion, and finger flexion of digits I to IV
- Numb and tingling-type paresthesias in digits I to IV and the palm
- Manifestations of complex regional pain syndrome may develop in the hand and forearm

Natural History

- Improves over months to about 1 year in cases due to penetrating trauma of elbow fractures
- Persistence in cases due to nerve compression by a supracondylar bone spur or entrapment in the region of the pronator teres unless the nerve is surgically decompressed

Diagnosis

Differential diagnosis

- Carpal tunnel syndrome
- Cervical radiculopathy involving the 6th or 7th nerve roots
- Upper or middle trunk brachial plexopathy
- Lateral or medial epicondylitis
- Focal manifestation of polyneuropathy, such as mononeuritis multiplex or multifocal motor neuropathy

History

- Abrupt onset of pain and sensory symptoms in the median territory and weakness of median supplied forearm and hand muscles during or shortly after venipuncture or arterial access procedures in the antecubital fossa, or in association with fractures in the elbow region
- Insidious onset of symptoms in lesions caused by compression at the supracondylar spur or within the pronator teres
- Production of or worsening of forearm pain and hand sensory symptoms during repeated or forceful forearm pronation when entrapment in the region of the pronator teres is the etiology
- Development of symptoms of causalgia (complex regional pain syndrome type II) after traumatic injuries

Physical examination

- Decreased sensation to light touch or pin prick in tips of digits I to IV and the palm
- Weakness of thumb abduction and opposition, wrist flexion, forearm pronation, and flexion of digits I to IV
- Atrophy of thenar and median supplied forearm muscles

- Local tenderness and Tinel's sign over the median nerve in the region of the elbow
- Reproduction of or worsening of forearm pain and hand sensory symptoms by resisted forearm pronation
- Allodynia and abnormalities of finger, hand, and distal forearm skin temperature if complex regional pain syndrome has developed

Testing

- Median nerve conduction studies, which show reduced amplitudes of the motor and sensory responses, normal motor and sensory distal latencies, and often mild slowing of the forearm conduction velocities
- Conduction studies in the adjacent nerves are normal unless polyneuropathy is present
- Needle EMG, which shows denervation in median supplied hand and forearm muscles
- Imaging of the elbow region to identify a supracondylar bony spicule of the distal humerus or fractures of the elbow

Treatment

- Analgesic and antineuropathic pain medications may improve neuropathic pain symptoms
- Surgical decompression when a supracondylar bony spur is present or when the diagnosis of pronator syndrome is made
- Appropriate and prompt management of complex regional pain syndrome if present

Prognosis

- Improvement over months to about 1 year in cases due to nerve trauma
- Improvement in sensory and motor symptoms over weeks to months in cases due to entrapment

Suggested Readings

Stevens JC. Median neuropathy. In: Dyck PJ, Thomas PK, eds. *Peripheral Neuropathy.* 4th ed. (pp. 1452–1454). Philadelphia, PA: Elsevier; 2005;

Stewart, John D. *Focal Peripheral Neuropathies* 4th ed. (pp. 200–207). West Vancouver, BC, Canada: JBJ Publishing; 2010.

Median Neuropathy—At the Wrist (Carpal Tunnel Syndrome)

John C. Kincaid MD

Description
Syndrome due to a focal lesion of the median nerve as it enters the hand

Etiology
- Entrapment of the median nerve as it enters the hand through the carpal tunnel
- Nerve trauma from penetrating injures or fractures of the distal forearm or wrist

Epidemiology
- Most common focal neuropathy
- Prevalence of 3% to 4% in the general population
- Three times more common in females
- 40 to 60 year age group more often affected
- Pregnancy

Pathogenesis
- Idiopathic cases are most common
- Exposure to vibrating hand tools, repetitive flexion/extension of the wrist and repetitive forceful hand grip
- Reduced tunnel dimensions due to arthritis of the wrist joint, ganglia, or congenital narrowing
- Generalized edema in mid-to-late pregnancy
- Infiltration of the tunnel by mucinous material in hypothyroidism or amyloid accumulation

Risk Factors
- Obesity
- Underlying polyneuropathy
- Vascular access creation for hemodialysis
- Pregnancy

Clinical Features
- Pain in the wrist and forearm
- Pain described as "deep in the bone"
- Tingling and/or numb-type paresthesias in the digits I to IV concurrent with the pain
- Improvement in the pain or paresthesias with change in hand position or shaking (flicking) the hand
- Symptoms usually begin in the dominant hand but commonly become bilateral
- Weakness of "pincher" motions involving digits I to IV
- Atrophy of thenar muscles in more severe cases
- Lesions due to penetrating trauma to the nerve often lack the nocturnal and position-related pain and sensory components

Natural History
- May improve over days to weeks with reduction in hand motion activities or after completion of pregnancy

Diagnosis

Differential diagnosis
- Arthritis involving the wrist or thumb
- Tendonitis of finger flexor or thumb extensor muscles
- Cervical radiculopathy involving the 6th or 7th nerve roots
- Upper or middle trunk brachial plexopathy
- Neurogenic thoracic outlet syndrome
- Proximal median neuropathy
- Focal manifestation of polyneuropathy

History
- Wrist or forearm pain, which worsens at night, while holding the hand on a steering wheel or during repetitive motion of the wrist or hand
- Sensory symptoms occurring in or worsening in the same setting as the pain
- Weakness of pincher motion of thumb-middle fingers

Physical examination
- Decreased sensation to light touch or pin prick in tips of digits I to IV in moderate-to-severe cases
- Two point discrimination threshold greater than 2 to 3 mm on tip of digits I to IV
- Weakness of thumb abduction and opposition in moderate-to-severe cases
- Atrophy of thenar muscles in moderate-to-severe cases
- Tinel's sign over the median nerve at the wrist
- Reproduction of or worsening of finger sensory symptoms by 10 to 30 seconds of wrist flexion (Phalen's sign)
- Flexion of distal thumb and tips of digits II to IV are normal

Testing

- Nerve conduction studies show prolongation of median distal latencies, sensory axons being affected earlier or more severely than motor
- Sensory and then motor response amplitudes become reduced in more severe cases
- Median motor and sensory conduction velocities in the forearm remain normal except in severe cases where mild slowing of motor velocity can be found
- Conduction studies in the adjacent nerves are normal unless polyneuropathy is present
- Needle EMG, which shows denervation in median supplied hand muscles in moderate-to-severe cases but median supplied forearm muscles as normal
- Ultrasound examination of the median nerve at the wrist in an emerging diagnostic tool whose ultimate role remains to be better defined

Treatment

- Analgesic, anti-inflammatory, and antineuropathic pain medications usually do not significantly improve the symptoms
- Reduce hand activity
- Improve ergonomics of hand, upper limb, and neck
- Wrist orthosis worn at night
- Steroid injection into the carpal tunnel if orthotic does not eliminate or greatly improve symptoms
- Surgical decompression of the carpal tunnel if orthosis or steroid injection does not eliminate or greatly improve symptoms

Prognosis

- Improvement after surgery, pain often fully relieved as soon as postoperative pain clears
- Improvement in sensory and motor symptoms may be delayed by weeks or months if persisting rather than transient deficits were present preoperatively or if any underlying polyneuropathy is present.

Suggested Readings

Jablecki CK, Andary MT, et al. Practice parameter: Electrodiagnostic studies in carpal tunnel syndrome. *Neurology.* 2002;58:1589–1952.

Stewart, John D. *Focal Peripheral Neuropathies.* 4th ed. (pp. 214–241). West Vancouver, BC, Canada: JBJ Publishing; 2010.

Musculocutaneous and Lateral Antebrachial Cutaneous Neuropathy

John C. Kincaid MD

Description
Syndrome due to focal lesion of the musculocutaneous nerve or its lateral antebrachial cutaneous branch

Etiology
- Compression of the nerve in shoulder dislocation or fracture of the proximal humerus
- Penetrating trauma by gun shot or stab wound
- Venipuncture in the lateral antecubital fossa
- Acute brachial plexitis
- Onset after vigorous elbow motions as in carrying heavy objects or pitching a ball

Epidemiology
- Rare lesion: occurs most often in association with shoulder dislocation or humeral fracture

Pathogenesis
- Demyelination and axonopathy due to compressive or penetrating lesions
- Inflammatory neuritis

Risk Factors
- Shoulder dislocation and proximal humeral fracture
- Venipuncture in the lateral antecubital fossa

Clinical Features
- Weakness of elbow flexion
- Sensory disturbance in the lateral aspect of the forearm

Natural History
- Improvement over several months to about 1 year

Diagnosis
Differential diagnosis
- Cervical radiculopathy involving the 5th or 6th nerve roots
- Brachial plexitis involving the upper trunk or lateral cord
- Biceps tendon rupture

History
- Weakness of elbow flexion, which is most often of abrupt onset and in association with trauma to the shoulder or proximal arm
- Sensory symptoms of the lateral forearm (occurs without motor dysfunction if only the lateral antecubital branch is involved)
- Shoulder and upper arm pain for several weeks and then onset of weakness if brachial plexitis is the etiology

Physical examination
- Weakness of elbow flexion and supination
- Atrophy of the biceps and brachialis muscles
- Impaired or absent biceps muscle stretch reflex
- Impaired cutaneous sensation over the lateral aspect of the forearm

Testing
- Needle EMG of the biceps, brachialis, and other muscles supplied by C5 and C6
- Sensory nerve conduction studies of the lateral antebrachial nerve looking for reduction in the amplitude or absence of the sensory action potential
- Motor conduction study of the nerve to the biceps looking for reduced amplitude of the compound muscle action potential. Comparison to the opposite side may be helpful in defining abnormality
- Radiographic studies of the shoulder and proximal humerus if the onset scenario suggests trauma
- Magnetic resonance imaging (MRI) of the cervical spine to evaluate the C5 and C6 spinal segments
- MRI of the brachial plexus looking for enhancement of the upper trunk or lateral cord

Treatment
■ Manage associated trauma of the shoulder or humerus
■ Physical medicine and physical therapy evaluations to optimize recovery of muscle function

Prognosis
■ Improvement in motor and sensory functions over several months to about 1 year after onset

Suggested Readings
Stewart, John D. *Focal Peripheral Neuropathies.* 4th ed. (pp 177–182). West Vancouver, BC, Canada: JBJ Publishing; 2010.
Wilbourn AJ, Ferrante MA. Upper limb neuropathies. In: Dyck PJ, Thomas PK, eds. *Peripheral Neuropathy.* 4th ed. (pp. 1471–1474). Philadelphia,PA: Elsevier; 2005.

Obturator Neuropathy

John C. Kincaid MD

Description
Syndrome due to a focal lesion of the obturator nerve

Etiology
- Nerve trauma due to intra-pelvic surgery
- Nerve trauma during fractures of the pelvis or hip
- Compression by intra-pelvic masses: neoplasm or endometriosis
- Compression during parturition: fetal head versus maternal positioning
- Entrapment in the obturator canal

Epidemiology
Rare lesion in isolation, much less common than femoral or sciatic neuropathy

Pathogenesis
- Local demyelination and in more severe lesions, axonopathy
- Inflammatory neuritis as a component of the lumbar plexitis syndrome

Risk Factors
- Intra-pelvic surgery
- Prolonged obstetric labor

Clinical Features
- Pain in the groin and upper medial thigh
- Weakness of hip adduction

Natural History
- May improve over weeks to months when a single episode of nerve compression is the etiology

Diagnosis

Differential diagnosis
- Arthritis of the hip joint
- Lumbar radiculopathy at the L1 or L2 level
- Lumbar plexopathy/plexitis

History
- Pain in the groin or medial, proximal thigh
- Instability/weakness in walking due to loss of adductor muscle power

Physical examination
- Weakness of leg adduction
- Sensory loss in the medial thigh

Testing
- Imaging of the pelvis to investigate the retroperitoneal and pericystic or perirectal area
- Imaging of the hip joint and bony pelvis
- Needle EMG of the adductor muscles and the quadriceps

Treatment
- Analgesic, anti-inflammatory and antineuropathic pain medications may partially improve symptoms
- Expectant observation over months if the lesion is associated with intra-pelvic surgery or delivery
- Manage endometriosis and other intra-pelvic lesions
- Diagnostic block of the obturator nerve
- Surgical decompression of the nerve in the obturator canal

Prognosis
- Improvement over weeks to months

Suggested Readings
Sorenson EJ, Chen JJ, Daube JR. Obturator neuropathy: Causes and outcome. *Muscle Nerve.* 2002;25:605–607.

Stewart, John D. *Focal Peripheral Neuropathies.* 4th ed. (pp. 568–573). West Vancouver, BC, Canada: JBJ Publishing; 2010.

Peroneal (Fibular) Neuropathy: Common, Deep, and Superficial Branch Lesions

John C. Kincaid MD

Description
Syndrome due to focal lesion of the peroneal nerve along its course from the knee to the ankle

Etiology
- Nerve trauma from traction, penetrating or lacerating injuries, or compression during fibular fracture
- Compression during repetitive leg crossing
- Entrapment in the region of the fibular head during repetitive or prolonged kneeling or squatting
- Compression by a ganglion cyst or benign nerve tumor
- Focal manifestation of a polyneuropathy such as mononeuritis multiplex or multifocal motor neuropathy

Epidemiology
Commonly encountered lesion, only lateral cutaneous neuropathy is a more common lower extremity lesion

Pathogenesis
- Compression, traction, or laceration of the nerve with resultant demyelination and axonopathy

Risk Factors
- Knee or lower leg trauma
- Repetitive leg crossing, particularly when associated with significant weight loss
- Surgical procedures on the knee

Clinical Features
- Lesions of the common peroneal nerve: weakness in ankle dorsiflexion, toe extension, and foot eversion along with tingling and/or numb-type paresthesias on the lateral aspect of the leg and dorsum of the foot
- Lesions of the deep branch of the nerve: weakness of ankle dorsiflexion and toe extension plus tingling and/or numb-type paresthesias of the web space between toes I and II but without weakness in foot eversion
- Lesions of the superficial branch of the nerve: weakness of foot eversion plus tingling and/or numb-type paresthesias on the distal lower leg and dorsum of the foot but without weakness in ankle dorsiflexion or toe extension

Natural History
- Abrupt onset when associated with trauma
- Insidious onset when associated with repetitive leg crossing or a compressive mass lesion such as a ganglion cyst

Diagnosis

Differential diagnosis
- Lumbar radiculopathy involving the 4th or 5th nerve root
- Lumbosacral plexopathy
- Sciatic neuropathy

History
- Weakness of ankle and toe extension producing foot drop or foot slap
- Numbness and tingling on the lower lateral leg and dorsum of the foot

Physical examination
- Weakness in ankle dorsiflexion, toe extension, and foot eversion, or a combination of these deficits, depending on the lesion location
- Atrophy of the muscles of the anterior compartment of the lower leg
- Sensory loss in the superficial and/or deep peroneal territories

Testing
- Peroneal motor nerve conduction studies can show reduction of compound muscle action potential (CMAP) amplitude from knee, fibular head, ankle, or a combination of these stimulation sites depending on the nature of the lesion. A low amplitude response from the knee but normal responses from the fibular head and ankle suggest a focal demyelinating-type lesion at the knee. Low amplitude responses at each of these sites indicate axon loss as the predominant pathology. Conduction velocities may be slow in the knee to ankle or knee to fibular head segments of the nerve. The motor distal latency should be normal. Motor conduction study to the tibialis anterior may be helpful if the study to the extensor digitorum brevis shows no measurable response. Sensory conduction study

of the superficial peroneal branch will be abnormal if the axons of this branch have been damaged but will be normal if conduction block at the knee is the predominant pathology.

- If axonal damage is present, the needle EMG will show denervation in peroneal supplied leg and foot muscles but will produce normal results in the short head of the biceps femoris and in nonperoneal supplied muscles. Needle EMG can also be helpful in determining the status of reinnervation after the initial lesion.
- Magnetic resonance imaging (MRI) of the knee region to define skeletal and soft tissue anatomy, especially when a causative lesion is not apparent
- Ultrasound examination of the nerve in the distal upper leg to fibular head region

Treatment

- Reduce or eliminate leg crossing at the knee and repetitive squatting or kneeling

- Ankle foot orthosis to stabilize ankle extensor/everter functions
- Surgical exploration of the nerve in the knee region if a mass lesion is seen on imaging studies
- Tendon transfer to correct persistent weakness of ankle extension

Prognosis

- Improvement over weeks to months after elimination of repetitive leg crossing or after surgical decompression if a mass lesion has been found
- Needle EMG can help define the status of reinnervation

Suggested Readings

Katirji B, Wilbourn A. Mononeuropathies of the lower limb. In: Dyck PJ, Thomas PK, eds. *Peripheral Neuropathy.* 4th ed. (pp. 1487–1510). Philadelphia, PA: Elsevier; 2005.

Stewart, John D. *Focal Peripheral Neuropathies.* 4th ed. (pp. 472–509). West Vancouver, BC, Canada: JBJ Publishing; 2010.

Phrenic Neuropathy

John C. Kincaid MD

Description
Syndrome due to a focal lesion of the phrenic nerve

Etiology
- Trauma to the nerve during cervical, cardiac, or other chest surgeries; during regional anesthesia involving the brachial plexus or jugular intravenous line placement
- Inflammatory neuritis as a component of brachial plexitis or Herpes Zoster involving the C3 to C5 levels
- Motor neuron disease predominantly involving the C3 to C5 segments of the spinal cord
- Infiltration by neoplasms

Epidemiology
Rare lesion except in the setting of cardiac surgery where the nerve may develop abnormal function in up to 10% of cases.

Pathogenesis
- Nerve trauma producing demyelination and axonal degeneration
- Autoimmune inflammatory neuritis

Risk Factors
Cardiac surgery

Clinical Features
- Orthopnea and dyspnea on exertion
- Pain in the neck or shoulder if the neuropathy is due to inflammatory neuritis
- Weakness in other territories of the upper brachial plexus if the phrenic neuropathy is a component of brachial plexitis/plexopathy

Natural History
- May improve over weeks to many months depending on the etiology

Diagnosis

Differential diagnosis
- Intrinsic lung lesion
- Trauma to the diaphragm or its tendons

History
- Orthopnea or dyspnea on exertion after surgical procedures in the chest or neck
- Difficulty weaning from ventilation after chest or neck surgeries
- Pain in the neck or shoulder if inflammatory neuritis is the etiology

Physical examination
- Neurologic examination will usually be normal
- Signs of accessory respiratory muscle activation may be present

Testing
- Chest radiography to evaluate for elevation of the diaphragm on the involved side
- Fluoroscopic evaluation of the diaphragm during inspiration/expiration
- Nerve conduction study of the phrenic nerve
- Needle EMG of shoulder/arm muscles if brachial plexitis/plexopathy is suspected
- Needle EMG of the diaphragm if the physician is competent in this technique

Treatment
- Expectant observation over months to about 2 years while reinnervation may occur
- Appropriate management of respiratory deficits: upright sleeping position, nocturnal positive airway pressure

Prognosis
- Requires 3 to 6 months of observation to determine if reinnervation will occur

Suggested Readings
Stewart, John D. *Focal Peripheral Neuropathies*. 4th ed. (pp. 88–91). West Vancouver, BC, Canada: JBJ Publishing; 2010.
Tsao BE, Ostrovskiy DA. Phrenic neuropathy due to neuralgic amyotrophy. *Neurology* 2006;66:1582–1584.

Pudendal Neuropathy

John C. Kincaid MD

Description
Syndrome due to a lesion of the pudendal nerve

Etiology
- Compression or irritation of the nerve by intra-pelvic lesions, such as endometriosis or neoplasm
- External compression of the nerve in the perineum by prolonged, localized weight bearing, such as bicycle riding
- Nerve trauma from penetration during therapeutic injections, by fractures of the pelvis, during surgery involving the pelvic floor, or during prolonged/recurrent labor

Epidemiology
- Rare lesion

Pathogenesis
- Local demyelination and axonopathy due to the primary lesion

Risk Factors
- Endometriosis
- Long-distance bicycling
- Surgical procedures involving the pelvic floor
- Multiparous state

Clinical Features
- Symptoms are most often unilateral
- Pain in the perineum
- Numbness and/or paresthesia in the perianal area, perineum, scrotum or labia, and shaft and head of the penis or clitoris
- Erectile and ejaculatory dysfunction

Natural History
- Lesions due to local pressure on the nerve, such as by long-distance bicycle riding, may improve over weeks to months after changing seating position or seat style

Diagnosis

Differential diagnosis
- Other pelvic lesions involving the sacral plexus, perivesicular, or perirectal areas
- Inguinal neuropathy

History
- Abrupt onset following trauma to the nerve
- Slow or insidious onset in lesions due to recurring external compression or intra-pelvic mass lesions

Physical examination
- Decreased sensation to light touch or pin prick in the perianal area, scrotum or labia, or along the shaft and tip of the penis or clitoris

Testing
- Pelvic examination by a knowledgeable practitioner to identify lesions of the perineum
- Pelvic imaging to identify mass lesions
- Electrodiagnostic evaluation [nerve conduction studies (NCS) and needle EMG] of the pelvic floor by a practitioner experienced in these techniques
- Diagnostic pudendal nerve block

Treatment
- Analgesic, anti-inflammatory, and antineuropathic pain medications may improve pain and paresthesias
- Alter seat angle or seat style if compression due to bicycle riding is the etiology
- Surgical decompression if an entrapment-type lesion is suspected

Prognosis
- Improvement may occur in weeks to months if a modifiable causation is present

Suggested Readings
Stav K, Dwyer PL, Roberts L. Pudenal neuralgia. Fact or fiction? *Obstet Gynecol Surv.* 2009;64:190–199.

Stewart, John D. *Focal Peripheral Neuropathies.* 4th ed. (pp. 457–460). West Vancouver, BC, Canada: JBJ Publishing; 2010.

Radial Neuropathy—In the Arm

John C. Kincaid MD

Description

Syndrome due to a focal lesion of the radial nerve distal to the shoulder up to the elbow segment of the nerve

Etiology

- Humeral fractures at the mid to mid-distal level
- Prolonged external compression of the nerve against the humerus during periods of impaired consciousness
- Trauma from intramuscular injections
- Compression from vigorous contraction of the triceps or external objects such as rifle slings

Epidemiology

Uncommon but classic peripheral nerve lesion

Pathogenesis

Local demyelination and axonopathy due to the primary lesion

Risk Factors

- Impaired responsiveness due to alcohol, sedating medication, excessive fatigue, or coma
- Underlying polyneuropathy such as hereditary neuropathy with liability to pressure palsy

Clinical Features

- Weakness of wrist and finger extension
- Sensory impairment in the superficial radial territory

Natural History

- Tends to improve over days to about 8 weeks when the pathogenesis is local demyelination producing conduction block
- Recovery time frame is much longer when axonal damage predominates

Diagnosis

Differential diagnosis

- Stroke producing upper motor neuron-type weakness
- C7 radiculopathy
- Middle trunk or posterior cord brachial plexopathy

History

- Abrupt onset of wrist and finger extension weakness during trauma to the upper arm or upon awakening from a prolonged period of excessive sedation
- Paresthesias and numbness over the dorsal forearm, distal radial forearm, and radial aspect of the hand

Physical examination

- Weakness of wrist and finger extension
- Impaired contraction of the brachioradialis
- "Pseudo" weakness of ulnar hand intrinsic muscles if the hand is not supported into a neutral flexion–extension position during ulnar hand muscle testing
- Normal triceps strength
- Normal triceps muscle stretch reflex
- Sensory loss over the dorsal forearm, distal radial forearm, and radial aspect of the hand

Testing

- Motor nerve conduction study of the radial nerve may show partial conduction block in the region of the spiral groove.
- The finding of a normal to near-normal radial compound action potential amplitude with stimulation distal to the lesion at the level of the elbow when performed for more than 5 days after onset suggests the lesion is predominantly due to local conduction block (neurapraxia/demyelination).
- A normal sensory action potential from the radial sensory branch obtained 5 to 10 days after the onset also supports the lesion being due to local conduction block at the site of the lesion.
- Low or absent motor or sensory response amplitudes from elbow level stimulation 10 to 14 days after onset suggests axonal damage as the predominant pathology.
- Needle EMG performed 3 to 4 weeks after onset can also help reveal the degree of any axonal damage: abundant fibrillation potentials and positive sharp waves indicate axonopathy.
- Repeat needle EMG at 2-month intervals after onset can help detect reinnervation and define prognosis when deficits have persisted beyond 6 to 8 weeks.
- Imaging of the nerve by magnetic resonance imaging (MRI) or ultrasound can help define the status of nerve continuity if fracture or penetrating injury was the etiology.

Treatment

- Physiatric and physical therapy evaluations to determine the optimal range-of-motion exercises and orthoses while strength deficits are present
- Antineuropathic pain medication, such as gabapentin or pregabalin, may help if bothersome paresthesias are present.
- Consider surgical exploration at 8 to 12 weeks if nerve conduction studies continue to show a pattern of complete axonotmesis and needle EMG shows no signs of beginning reinnervation.

Prognosis

- Good over 6 to 8 weeks if conduction block (neurapraxia) is suggested by nerve conduction studies
- Guarded if axonal damage (axonotmesis) is suggested by nerve conduction studies

Suggested Readings

Stewart, John D. *Focal Peripheral Neuropathies*. 4th ed. (pp. 315–347). West Vancouver, BC, Canada: JBJ Publishing; 2010.

Wilbourn AJ, Ferrante MA. Upper limb neuropathies. In: Dyck PJ, Thomas PK, eds. *Peripheral Neuropathy*. 4th ed. (pp. 1474–1478). Philadelphia, PA: Elsevier; 2005.

Radial Neuropathy—Posterior Interosseous Neuropathy

John C. Kincaid MD

Description
Syndrome due to a lesion of the posterior interosseous branch of the radial nerve

Etiology
- Entrapment of this branch of the radial nerve as it passes through the supinator muscle (Arcade of Frohse)
- Compression by lipoma, ganglia, or hypertrophied synovium
- Nerve trauma due to fracture of the proximal ulna or radius

Epidemiology
- Rare lesion, encountered about once every 2 years in an 1800-patient per year tertiary level electromyography (EMG) laboratory

Pathogenesis
- Demyelination and axonopathy due to compression of the nerve

Risk Factors
- Proximal fractures of the ulna or radius
- Repetitive vigorous pronation and supination

Clinical Features
- Weakness of finger extension, all fingers versus predominant weakness of the thumb, index, or middle fingers

Natural History
- May improve over days to weeks with reduction of forearm overuse
- More commonly the deficits persist until the nerve is surgically decompressed

Diagnosis

Differential diagnosis
- Lateral epicondylitis
- Cervical radiculopathy involving the 6th or 7th nerve roots with predominant involvement of finger extensors (pseudoposterior interosseous syndrome)
- Brachial plexitis with predominant involvement of axons to the finger extensors
- Proximal radial neuropathy
- Multifocal polyneuropathy: multifocal motor neuropathy or mononeuritis multiplex

History
- Spontaneous, insidious onset versus less common pattern of abrupt onset following vigorous, repetitive supination/pronation activities
- Variable pain component: proximal forearm or wrist location if present
- No sensory loss or paresthesia-type symptoms

Physical examination
- Weakness in extension of digits I to V: thumb, index, or middle fingers may be predominantly involved in some patients
- Atrophy of extensor digitorum communis may occur in longstanding cases
- A variable degree of tenderness along the course of the nerve in the region of the supinator (5–10 cm distal to the lateral epicondyle)
- Sensory examination in the posterior cutaneous nerve of the forearm and superficial radial nerve territories should be normal.

Testing
- Radial motor nerve conduction studies may show reduced amplitude of the compound muscle action potential recorded from the extensor digitorum communis or extensor indicis proprius as well as prolonged latency to those muscles with elbow-level nerve stimulation.
- Sensory responses in the superficial radial nerve should be normal.
- Conduction studies in the adjacent nerves should be normal unless polyneuropathy is present.

- Needle EMG shows denervation in radial supplied hand muscles distal to the supinator
- Imaging studies of the proximal radius and ulna if traumatic event has occurred (current or remote time frames)
- Imaging of the region of the supinator by ultrasound or magnetic resonance imaging (MRI) in idiopathic cases to evaluate for lesions such as ganglia or lipoma

Treatment

- Analgesic, anti-inflammatory, and antineuropathic pain medications usually do not significantly improve the symptoms
- Reduce forearm and hand use, particularly repetitive pronation/supination activities
- Surgical decompression of nerve through the region of the supinator if onset was gradual without a clear precipitating event or if no improvement has occurred after a 4 to 6 week period of observation after a causative event

Prognosis

- Improvement spontaneously or after surgical decompression in a time course partly definable based on the degree of denervation present in the needle EMG

Suggested Readings

Stewart, John D. *Focal Peripheral Neuropathies.* 4th ed. (pp. 314–347). West Vancouver, BC, Canada: JBJ Publishing; 2010.

Wilbourn AJ, Ferrante MA. Upper limb neuropathies. In: Dyck PJ, Thomas PK, eds. *Peripheral Neuropathy.* 4th ed. (pp. 1474–1478). Philadelphia, PA: Elsevier; 2005.

Radial Neuropathy–Superficial Radial Sensory Neuropathy

John C. Kincaid MD

Description

Syndrome due to a lesion of the superficial branch of the radial nerve

Etiology

- Direct compression by overly tight watch bands, handcuffs, or casts in the mid-to-distal forearm
- Nerve trauma from intravenous catheter insertion, during surgery in the distal forearm or wrist region or direct trauma during a fracture

Epidemiology

- Annual incidence is 0.003% in the general population

Pathogenesis

Local demyelination and axonopathy depending on the severity of the lesion.

Risk Factors

- Intravenous catheter insertion in the distal, radial forearm
- Surgical treatment of de Quervain's syndrome

Clinical Features

- Tingling and/or numb-type paresthesias in the distal, radial forearm and dorsum of the thumb, index, and middle digits
- Normal finger and wrist extensor strength in the finger and wrist extensor muscles

Natural History

- May improve over weeks to months

Diagnosis

Differential diagnosis

- Extensor tendonitis of the thumb (de Quervain's syndrome)
- Carpal tunnel syndrome
- Cervical radiculopathy involving the 5th or 6th nerve roots
- Upper trunk brachial plexopathy
- Proximal radial neuropathy
- Focal manifestation of multifocal polyneuropathy, such as mononeuritis multiplex

History

- Onset usually follows a definable event
- Distal forearm and dorsal hand paresthesias, which may worsen with wrist motions
- Cutaneous hypersensitivity in the area of the paresthesias

Physical examination

- Sensory deficits in the nerve's cutaneous area over the distal radial forearm and dorsum of the thumb, index, and middle digits
- Tinel's sign at the site of nerve compression
- Normal strength in finger and wrist extensor muscles

Testing

- Radial sensory conduction studies show reduced action potential amplitude or absence of a measurable response
- Radial motor conduction studies should be normal
- Conduction studies in adjacent nerves are normal unless polyneuropathy is present
- Needle EMG of the radial forearm and nonradial C5 or C6 muscles should be normal

Treatment

- Conservative observation over 4 to 12 week time course
- Antineuropathic pain medications may lessen the intensity of paresthesias and allodynia
- Treat concomitant conditions, such as de Quervain's tenosynovitis

Prognosis

- Improvement over weeks to months is expected but bothersome paresthesias and allodynia may persist for many months to years

Suggested Readings

Stewart, John D. *Focal Peripheral Neuropathies*. 4th ed. (pp. 315–347). West Vancouver, BC, Canada: JBJ Publishing; 2010.

Wilbourn AJ, Ferrante MA. Upper limb neuropathies. In: Dyck PJ, Thomas PK, eds. *Peripheral Neuropathy*. 4th ed. (pp. 1474–1478). Philadelphia, PA: Elsevier; 2005.

Sciatic Neuropathy

John C. Kincaid MD

Description

Syndrome due to a focal lesion of the sciatic nerve between the level of the piriformis muscle and the popliteal fossa

Etiology

- Nerve trauma due to pelvic or hip fracture, total hip arthroplasty, penetration by gun shots, stab wounds, or intramuscular injection
- Compression by hematoma or neoplasm
- Entrapment by the piriformis muscle

Epidemiology

- Occurs in about 1% of first time total hip replacement surgeries and up to about 5% of patients undergoing repeat procedures
- Rare lesion otherwise

Pathogenesis

Compression producing local demyelination and axonal damage

- Extraneural lesions are much more common
- Intraneural lesions such as peripheral nerve tumors are extremely rare

Risk Factors

- Total hip arthroplasty, especially revision procedures
- Fractures of the pelvis, hip, or femur
- Prolonged periods of unconsciousness or immobility
- Intramuscular injections into the gluteus maximus

Clinical Features

- Weakness in extensor and flexor motions of the ankle and toes
- Weakness of knee flexion may also be present
- Sensory deficits in the peroneal (fibular), posterior tibial, and sural territories
- Neuropathic pain in the foot and in some instances the entire leg
- Complex regional pain syndrome can occur in this setting

Natural History

- May improve over weeks to about 2 months in lesions that are predominantly demyelinating. Deficits can persist for many months or be permanent when axonal damage predominates

Diagnosis

Differential diagnosis

- Lumbar radiculopathy at the L5 or S1 level
- Lumbosacral plexopathy
- Arthritis of the hip joint
- Inflammation or instability of the sacroiliac joint

History

- Abrupt onset of symptoms shortly following trauma or at the time of awakening from surgery
- Indolent course in piriformis syndrome or intraneural neoplasm
- Weakness and pain tend to dominate the symptomatology
- Sensory deficits most commonly reported in the peroneal (fibular) territory

Physical examination

- Motor deficits in the peroneal (fibular) territory tend to be the more prominent: weakness of ankle extension and foot eversion
- Motor deficits in posterior tibial supplied muscle are often present but to a lesser degree: weakness of plantar flexion, foot inversion, toe flexion
- Depending on the location of the lesion knee, flexion may also be weak
- Ankle reflex is reduced or absent on the affected side
- Hip abduction and/or hip extension strength should be normal and the presence of weakness in these motions indicates that the lesion is in the sacral plexus or nerve root rather than the sciatic nerve
- Sensory deficits in the peroneal (fibular), posterior tibial, and sural nerve territories
- Reproduction of or worsening of sciatica by flexion-adduction-internal rotation-type maneuvers

Testing

- Motor nerve conduction studies should show reduced or absent compound muscle action potentials in the peroneal (fibular) and at times posterior tibial nerves. Conduction velocities tend to be mildly slow in an "axonal pattern" and distal latencies should remain normal. Focal slowing in the knee to fibular head segment of the peroneal nerve should not be present.

- Sensory conduction studies will show low amplitude or absent responses in the superficial peroneal and sural nerves if axon loss is a component of the lesion
- Peroneal and tibial nerve F-wave responses will be slowed or absent
- The H reflex may be slowed or absent depending on the degree of involvement of the posterior tibial nerve component
- Needle EMG will likely show signs of axonal damage in peroneal and to a lesser degree posterior tibial nerve territories. Gluteal muscles and the lumbar paraspinals should be normal if the lesion is at the sciatic nerve rather than the lumbosacral plexus or nerve root.
- Depending on the specific scenario, imaging studies of the hip joint, lumbar spine, pelvis, lumbosacral plexus, and proximal leg, including the piriformis muscle may be needed.

Treatment

- Analgesic and antineuropathic pain medications may significantly improve the symptoms
- Physical therapy to optimize function and facilitate recovery
- Ankle foot orthosis to stabilize foot drop
- Decompression of the nerve in the piriformis if a lesion at that site is supported by the evaluation

Prognosis

- Improvement over weeks to months in cases due to total hip arthroplasty, fractures of the femur, and penetrating injury

Suggested Readings

Katirji B, Wilbourn A. Mononeuropathies of the lower limb. In: Dyck PJ, Thomas PK, eds. *Peripheral Neuropathy*. 4th ed. (pp. 1487–1510). Philadelphia, PA: Elsevier; 2005.

Stewart, John D. *Focal Peripheral Neuropathies*. 4th ed. (pp. 432–471). West Vancouver, BC, Canada: JBJ Publishing; 2010.

Spinal Accessory Neuropathy

John C. Kincaid MD

Description
Syndrome due to a lesion of the spinal accessory nerve

Etiology
- Trauma to the nerve during radical nerve surgery or lymph node biopsy
- Blunt force and traction on the nerve in the setting of shoulder trauma
- Inflammation of the nerve as part of the brachial plexitis syndrome

Epidemiology
A lesion of this nerve occurs most often in the setting of surgery on the anterior lateral neck for treatment of cancer or as a complication of lymph node biopsy in the lower lateral neck.

Pathogenesis
- Demyelination and axonopathy secondary to the primary etiology
- Inflammatory neuritis

Risk Factors
- Cancer surgery on the neck
- Lymph node biopsy in the posterior-lateral neck

Clinical Features
- Weakness of shoulder motions
- Pain in the lower neck and top of the shoulder

Natural History
- May improve over months to about 1 year

Diagnosis

Differential diagnosis
- Cervical radiculopathy
- Arthritis of the shoulder
- Rotator cuff dysfunction
- Brachial plexopathy/plexitis
- Long thoracic neuropathy

History
- Weakness of shoulder shrug and abduction movements of the arm
- Pain in the upper shoulder and lateral neck
- Onset may follow a definable event such as surgery or may occur spontaneously

Physical examination
- Atrophy of trapezius: upper, middle, or lower components
- Muscle bulk and strength of sternomastoid muscle is normal unless the lesion is very proximal
- Scapular winging, more notable in arm abduction rather than protraction movements
- Normal cutaneous sensation unless adjacent sensory nerves are also affected: the lesser occipital and greater auricular nerves being the more likely to show deficits

Testing
- Nerve conduction studies of the spinal accessory nerve show reduction of compound muscle action potential (CMAP) amplitude on the affected side
- Needle EMG shows denervation in the upper, middle, or lower portions of the trapezius

Treatment
- Expectant observation over 3 to 6 months to determine if reinnervation will occur
- Cable grafting of the nerve when it must be sacrificed during radical surgery for cancer
- Physical therapy to improve shoulder motion and strength

Prognosis
- Improvement over months to about 1 year depending on the success of reinnervation

Suggested Readings
Stewart, John D. *Focal Peripheral Neuropathies*. 4th ed. (pp. 91–95). West Vancouver, BC, Canada: JBJ Publishing; 2010.

Kim DH, Cho YJ, Tiel Rl. Surgical outcomes of 111 spinal accessory nerve injuries. *Neurosurg*. 2003;53:1106–1112.

Suprascapular Neuropathy

John C. Kincaid MD

Description
- Syndrome due to a focal lesion of the suprascapular nerve

Etiology
- Entrapment in the region of the suprascapular notch on the superior aspect of the scapula or in the spinoglenoid notch as the nerve passes under the spine of the scapula
- Damage to the nerve in the setting of trauma to or dislocation of the shoulder
- Traction on the nerve at the level of the suprascapular notch in repetitive sports activities, such as baseball pitching or volleyball playing
- Focal manifestation of brachial plexitis

Epidemiology
Rare lesion

Pathogenesis
- Demyelination and axonopathy
- Inflammatory neuritis
- Compression from a shoulder cyst

Risk Factors
- Shoulder trauma
- Competitive baseball pitching or volleyball playing

Clinical Features
- Weakness in shoulder abduction and external rotation
- Weakness only in external rotation if the lesion is in the spinoglenoid notch
- Pain in the upper posterior shoulder area, may be absent in some patients
- No cutaneous sensory abnormalities

Natural History
- May improve over months if a specific etiology is identified and is corrected

Diagnosis
Differential diagnosis
- Lesion of the shoulder joint or associated muscular and tendon structures
- Cervical radiculopathy involving the 5th or 6th nerve roots
- Brachial plexopathy or plexitis with predominant involvement of the suprascapular nerve

History
- Weakness in shoulder abduction and external rotation motions
- Pain in the superior aspect of the shoulder (not present in all patients)

Physical examination
- Weakness in shoulder abduction and external rotation (only the latter may be present in some cases)
- Atrophy of supra- and infraspinatus muscles
- Normal strength and bulk of the deltoid, biceps, and serratus anterior muscles
- Pain in the superior shoulder region during resisted shoulder abduction or during palpation of the region of the suprascapular notch

Testing
- Needle EMG of muscles supplied by the upper trunk of the brachial plexus including the supra- and infraspinatus
- Nerve conduction study of the suprascapular nerve if the practitioner is skilled in this technique
- Magnetic resonance imaging (MRI) of the shoulder joint and associated soft tissue structures, including assessment of the size of the suprascapular notch; may see a cyst compressing the nerve
- Local anesthetic block at the suprascapular notch if pain is a significant component of the syndrome

Treatment
- Conservative observation if the lesion is due to shoulder trauma or is an isolated manifestation of brachial plexitis
- Appropriate management of degenerative lesions of the shoulder joint and associated soft tissue structures
- Reduction or modification of shoulder motions in lesions related to sports activities

■ Surgical decompression of the nerve at the suprascapular notch if local pain is a prominent manifestation and if local anesthetic block improves the pain

Prognosis

■ Improvement in strength over months

Suggested Readings

Antoniadis G, Richter HP. Suprascapular nerve entrapment: Experience with 28 cases. *J Neurosurg.* 1996; 85:1020–1025.

Stewart, John D. *Focal Peripheral Neuropathies.* 4th ed. (pp. 166–172). West Vancouver, BC, Canada: JBJ Publishing; 2010.

Tibial Neuropathy—In the Ankle and Foot

John C. Kincaid MD

Description

Syndrome due to a focal lesion of the distal portion of the tibial nerve

Etiology

- Nerve trauma due to fracture
- Entrapment in the tarsal tunnel
- Compression of the interdigital sensory branches at the metatarsal head (Morton's neuroma)

Epidemiology

Rare lesions, much less common than lesions of the sciatic or peroneal nerves

Pathogenesis

- External nerve trauma with resulting demyelination and axonal pathology
- Entrapment in potentially constricting spaces

Risk Factors

- Distal tibial fractures
- Arthritis of the ankle joint
- Wearing "overly fashionable" high heeled shoes

Clinical Features

- The lesion is predominantly unilateral

Ankle and proximal foot lesions

- Weakness of toe flexion and abduction
- Sensory loss in the medial, lateral, or both plantar nerve territories on the plantar surface of the foot
- Sensory loss over the plantar aspect of the heel

Interdigital nerve lesions (Morton's neuroma)

- Pain in region of the metatarsal head during weight bearing

Natural History

- May improve over weeks to many months after changes in activities involving the foot or change in shoe style

Diagnosis

Differential diagnosis

- Sciatic neuropathy
- S1 radiculopathy
- Sacral plexopathy
- Tibial neuropathy arising proximal to the ankle
- Polyneuropathy
- Plantar fasciitis or other soft tissue lesions of the foot

History

- Abrupt onset of motor and sensory deficits following traumatic lesions
- Gradual onset in compressive lesions within the tarsal tunnel or at the metatarsal head

Physical examination

Ankle and proximal foot lesions

- Weakness of toe flexion and abduction if the lesion is at the ankle
- Atrophy of tibial innervated foot muscles
- Normal ankle muscle stretch reflex
- Sensory loss in the territories of the medial plantar, lateral plantar, and calcaneal nerves or any combination of these if the lesion is at the ankle
- Sensory loss in two adjacent toes if the lesion is at the metatarsal head
- Tinel's sign from the nerve at the level of the medial malleolus or abductor hallucis
- Normal examination of the peroneal and saphenous nerves

Interdigital nerve lesions (Morton's neuroma)

- Reproduction of pain and/or paresthesia with deep palpation of the interdigital space, most often between the 3rd and 4th metatarsal heads, if the lesion is at the level of the interdigital nerve

Testing

Ankle and proximal foot lesions

- Tibial motor nerve conduction studies should show prolongation of the distal latency to the abductor hallucis and/or abductor digiti minimi pedis if the lesion is at the ankle. Compound muscle action potential (CMAP) amplitudes may be reduced if axon loss is also present. Conduction velocity in the knee to ankle segment should be normal unless significant axon loss is present.
- Mixed nerve conduction studies of the medial and lateral plantar nerves, if obtainable, may show prolongation of distal latency and loss of sensory nerve action potential (SNAP) amplitude.

- Conduction studies in the peroneal and sural nerves should be normal
- Needle EMG will likely show denervation in tibial supplied foot muscles but muscles proximal to the ankle should be normal
- Imaging studies of the ankle and foot to identify compressive lesions, such as ganglion cysts

Treatment

- Reduce or modify foot activities
- Change to more supportive, less "overly fashionable" shoes
- Steroid injection in the tarsal tunnel or symptomatic metatarsal head interspace
- Surgical decompression of the tarsal tunnel

- For Morton's neuroma excision of the neuroma (fibroma) of the symptomatic interdigital nerve if conservative treatments fail

Prognosis

- Improvement in sensory symptoms and motor signs over months with modification of foot activities or shoe styles, or after surgical decompression

Suggested Readings

Katirji B, Wilbourn A. Mononeuropathies of the lower limb. In: Dyck PJ, Thomas PK, eds. *Peripheral Neuropathy*. 4th ed. (pp. 1487–1510). Philadelphia, PA: Elsevier; 2005.

Stewart, John D. *Focal Peripheral Neuropathies*. 4th ed. (pp. 510–539). West Vancouver, BC, Canada: JBJ Publishing; 2010.

Tibial Neuropathy–From Knee to Ankle

John C. Kincaid MD

Description
Syndrome due to focal damage to the tibial nerve between the knee and the ankle level

Etiology
- Nerve trauma due to penetrating injury or fracture
- Compression by synovial cysts in the knee region
- Benign nerve tumor

Epidemiology
Rare, much less common than sciatic, peroneal, or femoral lesions

Pathogenesis
- External nerve trauma with resulting demyelination and axonal pathology
- Compromise of the vascular supply to the nerve

Risk Factors
- Trauma to the femur, knee, tibia, or associated soft tissue
- Surgical procedures on the knee
- Regional anesthesia procedures involving the sciatic nerve

Clinical Features
- Weakness of ankle flexion and foot inversion, weakness of toe flexion, and toe abduction
- Sensory loss in the sural nerve territory and plantar aspect of the foot, depending on the lesion site. Sural deficits indicate a lesion at or proximal to the knee
- Causalgia, complex regional pain syndrome type II, may develop in the setting of tibial nerve injury

Natural History
- May improve over weeks to many months, depending on the nature of and severity of the causative lesion

Diagnosis

Differential diagnosis
- Sciatic neuropathy
- L5 or S1 radiculopathy
- Lumbosacral plexopathy
- Tibial neuropathy at the ankle
- Focal manifestation of a multifocal polyneuropathy such as mononeuritis multiplex
- Rupture of the Achilles tendon
- Plantar fasciitis or other soft tissue lesions of the foot

History
- Abrupt onset of motor and sensory deficits following traumatic lesions
- Gradual onset in compressive lesions such as synovial cysts or intraneural tumors

Physical examination
- Weakness of ankle plantar flexion and foot inversion
- Weakness of toe flexion and abduction
- Atrophy of calf and tibial supplied intrinsic foot muscles
- Loss of or reduction of the ankle muscle stretch reflex
- Sensory loss in the sural territory and plantar aspect of the foot
- Signs of autonomic overactivity if causalgia is present

Testing
- Motor nerve conduction studies should show loss of compound muscle action potential (CMAP) amplitude at both the knee and ankle stimulation sites and mild slowing of conduction velocity (note that the CMAP amplitude may drop by up to 50% between the ankle and the knee stimulus sites in some normal individuals). The distal latency should remain normal.
- Sensory nerve conduction studies may show loss of sensory nerve action potential (SNAP) amplitude in the sural sensory study, depending on the lesion site.
- Conduction studies in adjacent nerves should be normal unless the lesion involves the distal sciatic nerve, peroneal nerve concurrently, or if polyneuropathy is present.
- Needle EMG should show denervation in tibial supplied muscles of the lower leg and foot. Tibial innervated hamstring muscles and peroneal supplied muscles should be normal.

Treatment
- Analgesic and antineuropathic pain medications may improve symptoms
- Appropriate management if causalgia, complex regional pain syndrome type II, is present
- Physical therapy to maximize functional recovery
- Surgical exploration and decompression if a mass lesion is the etiology

Prognosis

- Improvement in sensory and motor deficits over months to about 2 years depending on the severity of the causative lesion.

Suggested Readings

Katirji B, Wilbourn A. Mononeuropathies of the lower limb. In: Dyck PJ, Thomas PK, eds. *Peripheral Neuropathy*. 4th ed. (pp. 1500–1503). Philadelphia, PA: Elsevier; 2005.

Stewart, John D. *Focal Peripheral Neuropathies*. 4th ed. (pp. 510–539). West Vancouver, BC, Canada: JBJ Publishing; 2010.

Trigeminal Neuralgia and Neuropathy

John C. Kincaid MD

Description

Syndromes due to lesions of the trigeminal nerve

- Trigeminal neuralgia (tic douloureux) manifests as recurrent unilateral short-lived paroxysms of severe facial pain
- Trigeminal neuropathy manifests as loss of sensation, often without a painful component

Etiology

Trigeminal neuralgia

- Compression of the sensory root of the nerve proximal to the Gasserian ganglion by branches of the superior cerebellar artery
- Inflammatory demyelination of the sensory axons within the brainstem due to multiple sclerosis
- Idiopathic

Trigeminal neuropathy

- Nerve trauma due to facial or mandibular fractures, dental extractions, or skull base surgery
- Compression or invasion of the nerve by skull base or nasopharyngeal neoplasms
- Local inflammation of the nerve due to Herpes Zoster attacks or connective tissue diseases, such as scleroderma or mixed connective tissue disease
- Idiopathic

Epidemiology

- Trigeminal neuralgia's annual incidence is 4 to 25 cases per 100,000 of population with higher incidence occurring in older individuals
- Trigeminal neuropathies are much less common than trigeminal neuralgia

Pathogenesis

- Trigeminal neuralgia: local demyelination of the peripheral or central trigeminal sensory axons allows spontaneous generation of action potentials in nociceptive neurons
- Trigeminal neuropathy: local demyelination and axonal damage due to trauma, compression, or inflammation of trigeminal sensory axons and at times motor axons

Risk Factors

- Facial trauma
- Dental extractions
- Multiple sclerosis, particularly in trigeminal neuropathy patients with onset below age
- 50 years
- Herpes Zoster involving the trigeminal nerve

Clinical Features

Trigeminal neuralgia

- Unilateral paroxysms of intense "electric"- or "hot poker"-like pain lasting seconds
- Pain is often provoked by facial or jaw movement or cutaneous stimulation within the trigeminal sensory territory
- Attacks tend to not occur during sleep
- The second or third divisions of the nerve are more often affected
- Absence of persisting sensory loss in the affected division of the nerve

Trigeminal neuropathy

- Unilateral loss of sensation in the trigeminal territory
- Pain is a less common feature except in cases occurring as component of a Herpes Zoster attack
- Motor deficits can occur if the mandibular division is involved

Natural History

- Trigeminal neuralgia: recurring attacks of pain, although spontaneous remissions can occur
- Trigeminal neuropathy: persistent sensory deficits

Diagnosis

Differential diagnosis

- Trigeminal neuralgia: migraine headache, cluster headache, temporomandibular joint dysfunction, sinusitis, and dental disease
- Trigeminal neuropathy: brainstem infarction, sinusitis, and facial trauma

History
- Trigeminal neuralgia: paroxysmal unilateral short-lived attacks of intense electric jabbing pain in the forehead, maxilla, or mandible often provoked by face or jaw movements
- Trigeminal neuropathy: persistent sensory loss in the territory of the trigeminal nerve

Physical examination

Trigeminal neuralgia
- Normal sensory and motor functions of the trigeminal and adjacent cranial nerve territories
- An attack of pain may be provoked by cutaneous stimuli in the affected division of the nerve

Trigeminal neuropathy
- Loss of sensation in the affected division(s) of the nerve
- Atrophy of the masseter and temporalis muscles may be present if the mandibular division is involved

Both conditions: absence of jaw crepitance during opening/closing motions.

Testing
- Imaging of the brain stem and course of the trigeminal nerve through the skull base
- Imaging of the sinuses
- Connective tissue disease serologies: ANA, SS-A, and SS-B
- Dental examination
- Blink reflex testing for trigeminal neuropathy

Treatment

Trigeminal neuralgia
- Antiepileptic medications: carbamazepine or oxcarbazine
- Gabapentin and baclofen can be used as adjunctive medications
- Surgical decompression of the sensory root if medical treatment fails
- Gamma-knife treatment is also a viable option for patients not fully responsive to medical management
- Rhizotomy of the Gasserian ganglion by thermal or chemical means

Trigeminal neuropathy
- Antibiotics for sinusitis
- Antibiotic and surgical management of dental infection
- Immune suppressive/modulation for connective tissue disease
- Appropriate management of Herpes Zoster attack and postherpetic neuralgia

Prognosis
- The pain of trigeminal neuralgia should be fully controllable in the vast majority of patients by medical or surgical means
- The sensory loss due to trigeminal neuropathy tends to persist

Suggested Readings
Hughes R. Diseases of the fifth cranial nerve. In: Dyck PJ, Thomas PK, eds. *Peripheral Neuropathy.* 4th ed. (pp. 1207–1217). Philadelphia, PA: Elsevier; 2005.
Love S, Coakham H. Trigeminal neuralgia, pathology and pathogenesis. *Brain* 2001;124:2347–2360.

Ulnar Neuropathy—At the Elbow

John C. Kincaid MD

Description
Syndrome due to a lesion of the ulnar nerve in the region of the elbow

Etiology
- Entrapment by the proximal aspect of the flexor carpi ulnaris (cubital tunnel retinaculum) during elbow flexion
- Compression of the nerve just proximal to the medial epicondyle during prolonged or repetitive flexion (retro-epicondylar region)
- Entrapment due to osteoarthritis of the elbow joint years to decades after an elbow fracture (tardy ulnar palsy)
- Compression of the nerve during fracture of the distal humerus or proximal ulnar
- Lacerations of the nerve due to penetrating injury eg, glass shards, knife wounds
- Compression of the nerve during or immediately following surgery (intraoperative ulnar neuropathy)

Epidemiology
- Second most common entrapment mononeuropathy after carpal tunnel syndrome
- Seen more commonly in men

Pathogenesis
Local demyelination and then axonopathy, depending on the severity of the nerve compression

Risk Factors
- Prior elbow fracture with residual mal-alignment of the humerus and ulna (tardy ulnar palsy)
- Surgical procedures (intraoperative ulnar neuropathy)

Clinical Features
- Tingling and/or numb-type paresthesias in digits IV to V
- Pain in the medial elbow
- Weakness in ulnar-supplied hand and forearm muscles

Natural History
- May improve over days to weeks with reduction of repeated or prolonged periods of elbow flexion

Diagnosis

Differential diagnosis
- Medial epicondylitis
- Degenerative arthritis of the elbow
- Cervical radiculopathy involving the C8 or T1 nerve roots
- Lower trunk or medial cord brachial plexopathy
- Neurogenic thoracic outlet syndrome
- Ulnar neuropathy at the wrist
- Focal manifestation of polyneuropathy

History
- Paresthesias in digits IV to V, which worsens during elbow flexion
- Pain in the medial elbow region
- Weakness in fine motions of the digits or hand (eg, page turning, finger nail clipping, buttoning)

Physical examination
- Decreased sensation to light touch or pin prick in digits IV to V
- Decreased sensation to light touch or pin prick over the medial aspect of both the palmar and dorsal aspects of the hand
- Two point discrimination threshold greater than 2 to 3 mm on tip of digits IV to V
- Weakness of abduction and adduction of ulnar-supplied hand muscles
- Weakness of flexion of the distal interphalangeal joints of digits IV to V
- Atrophy of ulnar-supplied hand and medial forearm muscles in severe cases
- Subluxation of the nerve over the medial epicondyle during elbow flexion (occurs in ~20% of normal individuals)
- Tinel's sign along the nerve around the elbow
- Reproduction of or worsening of sensory symptoms by 30 seconds of full elbow flexion (elbow flexion test)
- Normal strength in non-ulnar C8 muscles, such as the abductor pollicis brevis and extensor pollicis longus

Testing
- Motor nerve conduction studies show slowing of conduction velocity in the elbow segment with normal velocity in the forearm. Distal latency should remain normal.

- In more severe cases that produce axon loss, the forearm conduction velocity may also be slow and the response amplitudes become reduced at stimulus sites both proximal and distal to the elbow
- Sensory responses from the fifth digit or the dorsal cutaneous branch will show reduced amplitudes with stimulation at the wrist when axonal damage is present
- Sensory responses from wrist-level stimulation will remain normal if the elbow lesion is predominantly demyelinating
- Median motor and sensory and radial sensory conduction studies should remain normal unless an underlying polyneuropathy is present
- When the lesion causes axonal damage, needle EMG will show abnormal resting activity and neurogenic-type motor unit potentials in ulnar-supplied hand and, in most instances, ulnar-supplied forearm muscles but should be normal in non-ulnar C8- or T1-supplied muscles.

Treatment

- Limit elbow flexion voluntarily or via an elbow pad, which secondarily impairs full elbow flexion
- Occupational therapy evaluation for padding and splinting of the elbow

- Observe the clinical status over 4 to 8 weeks and if improvement occurs, continue conservative treatment
- If symptoms persist or worsen during conservative treatment, refer the patient for surgical consultation: The surgical procedure may be decompression at the level of the proximal flexor carpi ulnaris or anterior submuscular transposition of the nerve.
- Ulnar neuropathy occurring in the intraoperative or immediately postoperative setting tends to respond less well to surgical intervention

Prognosis

- Improvement over weeks to 2 months with conservative treatment if the lesion is predominantly demyelinating
- Improvement over weeks if surgery is performed for patients not responding to conservative treatment
- Improvement over months in patients showing predominantly axonal-type abnormalities on preoperative electrodiagnostic studies

Suggested Readings

Campbell WW, Carroll DJ, et al. Practice parameter for electrodiagnostic studies in ulnar neuropathy at the elbow. *Muscle Nerve.* 1999;22:408–411.

Stewart, John D. *Focal Peripheral Neuropathies.* 4th ed. (pp. 260–313). West Vancouver, BC, Canada: JBJ Publishing; 2010.

Ulnar Neuropathy—At the Wrist

John C. Kincaid MD

Description
- Syndrome due to lesion of the ulnar nerve as it enters the hand (Guyon's canal)

Etiology
- Nerve trauma from recurring or sustained external pressure on the ulnar side of the hand
- Compression by ganglia, synovial cysts, and benign neoplasms

Epidemiology
Rare lesion: encountered approximately once in 5 years in an 1800-patient study per year tertiary level electromyography (EMG) laboratory

Pathogenesis
- Compression of the ulnar nerve in the "Guyon's canal" region of the hand

Risk Factors
- Long-distance cycling on a "ram's horn" handlebar type bicycle
- Use of the ulnar side of the heel of the hand as a "hammer"
- Prolonged or recurrent leaning on the base of the hand

Clinical Features
- Weakness of the ulnar innervated hand muscles
- Sensory loss in digits IV and V with sparing of the palmar and dorsal ulnar sensory areas of the hand
- Depending on the lesion site as the nerve enters the hand, four different clinical patterns may occur:
  - Weakness of all ulnar innervated hand muscles and abnormal sensation in digits IV to V;
  - Weakness in both hypothenar and ulnar intrinsic hand muscles with normal sensation;
  - Weakness in ulnar intrinsic hand but not hypothenar muscles with normal sensation (most common pattern); and
  - Sensory loss in digits IV to V with normal function of ulnar supplied hand muscles

Natural History
- May improve over weeks to months with reduction of the causative activity

Diagnosis

Differential diagnosis
- Ulnar neuropathy at the elbow
- C8 or T1 radiculopathy
- Lower trunk brachial plexopathy, including neurogenic thoracic outlet syndrome
- Arthritis or other bony abnormality of the wrist
- Tendinitis/tendinopathy of the ulnar aspect of the wrist/hand

History
- Weakness of ulnar-controlled finger motions
- Abnormal sensation in IV and V digits
- Hand or forearm pain is not a common feature

Physical examination
- Weakness of ulnar innervated hand muscles: hypothenar and intrinsic or intrinsic only
- Atrophy of ulnar innervated muscles in moderate-to-severe cases
- Normal function of flexor digitorum profundus and flexor carpi ulnaris muscles
- Normal function of median and radial innervated muscles of the hand and digits
- Decreased sensation to light touch or pin prick of the palmar aspect of digits IV to V
- Normal sensation over the ulnar area of the palmar and dorsal ulnar area of the hand
- Tinel's sign over the ulnar nerve at the wrist
- Inspect/palpate ulnar aspect of the wrist for mass lesion

Testing
- Ulnar motor conduction studies, including distal latency to the first dorsal interosseous muscle:
  - Lesions of the ulnar nerve at the wrist should produce prolongation of motor distal latency to the hypothenar muscles and/or first dorsal interosseous muscle depending on the exact lesion site at the wrist
  - Forearm and across-elbow conduction velocities should be normal

- Ulnar sensory conduction studies to the fifth digit and the dorsal cutaneous branch
- Median motor conduction study to evaluate for abnormalities in non-ulnar C8/lower trunk plexus supplied muscles
- Needle EMG of ulnar innervated hand and forearm muscles and median supplied thenar muscles
- Imaging of the hand by plain x-ray for fracture and by magnetic resonance imaging (MRI) or ultrasound for soft tissue-type lesions

Treatment

- Reduce activities that produce pressure on the ulnar aspect of the base of the hand
- Pad the base of the hand for activities such as bicycling

- Surgical exploration/decompression of the nerve if improvement of function does not occur over several months of observation or if a space occupying lesion is found on imaging studies

Prognosis

- Improvement over weeks to months after elimination of external compressive activities or surgical excision of space occupying lesions

Suggested Readings

Stewart, John D. *Focal Peripheral Neuropathies*. 4th ed. (pp. 297–313). West Vancouver, BC, Canada: JBJ Publishing; 2010.

Wu J-S, Morris JD, Hogan GR. Ulnar neuropathy at the wrist: Case report and review of literature. *Arch Phys Med Rehabil*. 1985;66:785–788.

Vagal (Laryngeal) Neuropathy

John C. Kincaid MD

Description
Syndromes due to lesions of the vagal nerve

- Abnormalities of laryngeal function: voice and laryngeal sensation
- Abnormalities of vagal autonomic function: heart rate regulation and gastrointestinal motility modulation

Etiology
- Nerve trauma, more commonly unilateral, during surgical procedures on thyroid, cervical spine, carotid artery, or skull base
- Nerve trauma during intrathoracic surgical procedures or during endotracheal intubation
- Compression or infiltration of the nerve by neoplasms in the neck or chest
- Idiopathic but presumably autoimmune inflammatory neuritis
- Local manifestation of generalized polyneuropathy

Epidemiology
Rare lesions except in the postoperative setting: temporary paresis occurs in 2% to 12% of thyroidectomies, 2% to 6% of carotid endarterectomies, and 2% of cervical spine surgeries done by the anterior approach

Pathogenesis
- Local demyelination and axonal damage secondary to compression or traction during surgery
- Nerve compression secondary to infiltration by neoplasms in the neck, or check along the course of the nerve
- Autoimmune inflammation of the nerve
- Axonopathy and demyelination due to an underlying polyneuropathy

Risk Factors
- Surgery on the neck, cervical spine, or intrathoracic structures
- Endotracheal intubation
- Malignancy of the thyroid or chest along the course of the nerve
- Presence of generalized polyneuropathy, such as Charcot-Marie-Tooth disease or diabetic neuropathy

Clinical Features
- Hoarseness and impaired ability to increase the volume of the voice
- Impairment raising the pitch of the voice
- Persistent cough
- Stridor when bilateral lesions are present
- Syncope or enhanced tendency for syncope

Natural History
Improvement in the majority of patients over several weeks to about 6 month time frame

Diagnosis

Differential diagnosis
- Central nervous system lesion of the lateral brainstem producing vagal dysfunction along with other signs, such as cerebellar ataxia and hemisensory loss
- Dislocation of the arytenoid bone during trauma to the larynx

History
- Abrupt onset of voice dysfunction in patients due to nerve trauma during a surgery
- Gradual onset and progressive voice dysfunction in patients due to compression or infiltration of the nerve by neck or thoracic neoplasms
- Persistent cough
- Enhanced tendency for syncope

Physical examination
- Dysphonia of a hoarse, raspy nature
- Impairment of vocal cord motion (requires visualization of the vocal cord)
- Findings of lateral medullary syndrome (unilateral lower limb ataxia and impairment of pain and temperature sensation along with vagal dysfunction)

Testing
- Evaluation of vocal cord function by laryngoscopy
- Imaging of neck and chest to identify mass lesions along the course of the vagal nerve
- Needle EMG of laryngeal muscles: abnormalities in both the cricothyroid and thyroarytenoid indicate a lesion of the nerve proximal to the bifurcation of the superior and recurrent laryngeal branches

- Assessment of swallowing function if dysphagia is a manifestation of the dysfunction
- Cardiac evaluation if new-onset syncope is a feature of the lesion
- Neurological evaluation if generalized neuropathy, features of basal ganglia disease, or motor neuron disease are present

Treatment

- Tracheostomy may be required if airway compromise occurs due to bilateral lesions, which leave the vocal cords in an adducted position
- Expectant observation over 3 to 6 months watching for recovery of nerve function

- Several surgical procedures are available to partially improve long-term vocal cord dysfunction
- Reinnervation phenomena such as spastic dysphonia can be treated by botulinum toxin injection into the thyroarytenoid muscle

Prognosis

Most patients improve over 3 to 6 months

Suggested Readings

Rosenthal L, Benninger M. Vocal fold immobility: A longitudinal analysis of etiology over 20 years. *Laryngoscope* 2007;117: 1864–1870.

Thomas P, Mathias C. Diseases of the ninth, tenth, eleventh and twelfth cranial nerves. In: Dyck PJ, Thomas PK, eds. *Peripheral Neuropathy*. 4th ed. (pp. 1273–1293). Philadelphia, PA: Elsevier; 2005.

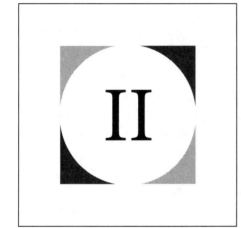

Polyneuropathies

Acute Inflammatory Demyelinating Polyradiculoneuropathy (Guillain-Barré Syndrome)

John C. Kincaid MD

Description
Acquired, autoimmune polyneuropathy, which reaches maximum clinical deficit over a time course of 8 weeks or less

Etiology
Autoimmune process, which attacks the myelin sheath and axons of the nerve roots and peripheral nerve trunks

Epidemiology
Prevalence of one case per 100,000 population

Pathogenesis
- Cellular rather than antibody-mediated autoimmune response, which cross reacts with antigens on the peripheral myelin sheath or axons of the nerve roots and nerve trunks
- Recent infection with *Campylobacter jejuni* (*C. jejuni*) is a potentially provoking factor in approximately 30% of cases
- Other cases may follow nonspecific respiratory infections, initial HIV infection, vaccination, or surgical procedures with a typical interval of 8 to 12 weeks or less between those events and the onset of the neuropathy

Risk Factors
- *C. jejuni* infection
- Vaccination against seasonal influenza

Clinical Features
- "Ascending" (distal to proximal, lower extremity somewhat earlier than upper extremity) pattern of motor and sensory deficits, with motor dysfunction usually being the more prominent feature
- Maximum deficit is reached by 8 weeks or less after onset, with 4 weeks or less being more typical
- Loss of muscle stretch reflexes
- Neuropathic pain in the limbs may occur but is usually not a prominent feature
- Sensations of band-like tightness may be experienced in truncal areas
- Autonomic dysfunction manifesting as unstable blood pressure or cardiac arrhythmias may occur
- Urinary and rectal sphincter functions usually remain normal

Natural History
- Improves over 3 to 12 months in most patients
- Severe persisting deficits occur in 5% to 10%

Diagnosis

Differential diagnosis
- Acute polyneuropathy due to other causes such as porphyria; adverse effects of medication such as cancer chemotherapy, nitrofurantoin, or metronidazole exposure, and/or arsenic poisoning
- Spinal cord lesion due to an inflammatory process such as transverse myelitis or the initial attack of multiple sclerosis
- Spinal cord compression due to spondylotic myelopathy
- Spinal cord infarction
- Poliomyelitis
- West Nile virus infection

History
- Paresthesias begin in the feet and spread proximally into the feet, legs, and upper extremities in a time course extending over several days to a maximum of 8 weeks
- Weakness evolves in the same distal to proximal, lower and upper extremity pattern described in clinical features
- Neuropathic pain tends to be a less prominent feature, but some patients report a "tight" or constrictive pattern in the thoracic/abdominal spinal areas

Physical examination
- Symmetrical weakness in distal and proximal muscles of the lower and upper extremities

- Weakness of facial muscles occurs in up to 50% and extraocular muscles may be affected in 5% to 10% of patients
- Respiratory failure due to pharyngeal, diaphragmatic, or chest wall muscle weakness occurs in 30% of patients
- Loss of muscle stretch reflexes
- Deficits in sensory function such as light touch, vibration, and pin prick sensation

Testing

- Motor nerve conduction studies show prolongation of distal latencies and slowing of conduction velocities in the forearm and leg segments of the nerves.
- Distal latencies greater than 125% of the upper limit of normal, conduction velocities less than 70% of the low limit of normal and conduction block with response amplitudes, dropping by more than 20% between proximal and distal stimulus sites support the neuropathy being predominantly demyelinating
- Sensory conduction studies also become abnormal by showing prolonged distal latencies and reduction of response amplitudes but nerves that do not pass through potential entrapments sites such as the sural and superficial radial may remain normal.
- The latencies of the F-wave and H-reflex become prolonged if they are recordable
- Needle EMG shows reduction of motor unit potential recruitment as the weakness begins and then may show fibrillations and positive waves by 4 to 8 weeks after onset, reflecting the development of axonal dysfunction
- Cerebrospinal fluid (CSF) analysis for protein and cell count
- Consider porphyria screen and urine arsenic level

Treatment

- Immune modulating therapy by plasma exchange or intravenous infusion of gamma-globulin shortens the duration of the deficits by 30% to 50%.
- Corticosteroids by oral or intravenous routes do not have any beneficial affect.

Prognosis

- Improvement over a 2- to 12-month time frame
- 10% of patients may have a partial relapse after an initial period of improvement
- 15% of patients are left with clinically significant deficits

Suggested Readings

Amato A, Russell J. *Neuromuscular Disorders* (pp 214–232). McGraw Hill, New York; 2008.

Griffin J, Sheikh K. The Guillain-Barré Syndromes. In: Dyck PJ, Thomas PK, eds. *Peripheral Neuropathy*. 4th ed. (pp. 2197–2219). Philadelphia, PA: Elsevier; 2005.

Amyloid Neuropathies

John C. Kincaid MD

Description

Peripheral neuropathies due to accumulation of specific proteins, which have a propensity to form insoluble extracellular fibrils in certain tissues

Etiology

The neuropathy occurs in two different settings:

- Sporadic (primary amyloid neuropathy) due to overproduction and tissue deposition of the light chain component of immunoglobulin
- Inherited (familial amyloid neuropathy) cases due to altered structure of a constituent protein resulting in an enhanced tendency for tissue deposition

Epidemiology

Neuropathies due to amyloidosis are rare:

- Sporadic cases are the more common type of a myloidosis and occur in the setting of a lymphoproliferative disorder
- Inherited cases show a dominant inheritance pattern

Pathogenesis

Overproduction of normal proteins, such as the gamma-light chain component of immunoglobulin, or alteration of the usual amino acid sequence of a constitutive protein, such as prealbumin (transthyretin), cause the protein to be less soluble than normal and to have an increased tendency to form deposits of a beta-sheet structure in certain tissues, including the peripheral nerves.

Clinical Features

- Onset of deficits in the 30- to 50-year-old age group is typical
- Gradual onset of sensory loss and paresthesia, beginning in the toes and feet is the more common pattern; lower extremity motor deficits may develop later as can hand sensory and motor deficits
- Carpal tunnel syndrome can be the initial presentation in some forms of amyloid neuropathy with polyneuropathy developing years later
- Autonomic, cardiac, renal, and hematologic dysfunction occurs in some forms of amyloidosis

Natural History

Gradual progression of the neuropathic and other organ deficits:

- Neuropathic deficits in the inherited forms may progress to a disabling degree
- Hematologic, cardiac, and renal deficits may progress to a severe degree

Diagnosis

Differential diagnosis

- Chronic inflammatory neuropathy
- Idiopathic carpal tunnel syndrome followed some years later by polyneuropathy due to another cause
- Other dominantly inherited polyneuropathies

History

- Sensory loss and paresthesias, beginning in feet
- Small fiber sensory functions, such as pain and temperature, may be predominantly affected early on in some inherited varieties with large fiber-type dysfunction occurring later
- Carpal tunnel syndrome is the initial manifestation in some types of amyloidosis
- Distal weakness usually occurs after sensory dysfunction
- Autonomic dysfunction manifesting as impotence, diarrhea, sphincter dysfunction, orthostatic hypotension, and impaired sweating are features of some forms

Physical examination

- Deficits in the sensory modalities of pin prick and temperature, light touch, vibration, and position sensation are the earliest findings in patients with polyneuropathy
- Sensory deficits and signs of nerve irritability in the median nerve territory may be found in patients with carpal tunnel syndrome as an early manifestation
- Symmetrical distal weakness of the lower and later the upper extremities
- Loss of muscle stretch reflexes consistent with the pattern of weakness
- Impaired pupillary reaction to light and orthostatic hypotension if autonomic functions are impaired
- Purpuric skin lesions

Testing

- Serum and urine protein electrophoresis to evaluate for the presence of a monoclonal protein or excessive production of gamma-light chains
- Bone marrow examination in patients with the primary form of amyloidosis
- Biopsy of abdominal fat pad, rectal mucosa, or peripheral nerve for demonstration of deposits, which stain with the dye Congo Red and show pink to green color change when viewed under polarized light
- Nerve conduction studies show an "axonal" pattern of abnormality: motor and sensory response amplitudes are low, conduction velocities are no slower than the mid-30 meter per second range, and distal latencies remain normal except in the median nerve
- Depending on the type of amyloid neuropathy, nerve conduction studies may show findings typical of median neuropathy at the wrist initially and polyneuropathy-type findings appear years later
- Cerebrospinal fluid values tend to be normal
- Electrocardiogram and echocardiogram to evaluate cardiac conduction and contractile functions

Treatment

- Symptomatic treatment for neuropathic pain
- Treat cardiac arrhythmias and heart failure

- Immune modulation with melphalan and steroids or high-dose melphalan followed by autologous stem cell rescue in primary amyloidosis
- Liver transplantation in Familial Amyloid Neuropathy may stabilize the peripheral nerve and cardiac components
- Treatment with protein-stabilizing agents such as difunisal and tamifidis (the latter is not available in the United States currently) may stabilize the neuropathy
- Down regulation of amyloid protein production by ribonucleic acid (RNA) interference mechanisms is being investigated in familial amyloidosis

Prognosis

- Hematologic, cardiac, and peripheral nerve components of primary amyloid may stabilize with treatment
- Peripheral nerve and cardiac components of familial amyloidosis may stabilize with treatment
- The role of emerging therapies such as protein-stabilizing medications and RNA interference modulation of production of the abnormal proteins remains to be more fully established.

Suggested Readings

Benson M, Kincaid J. The molecular biology and clinical features of amyloid neuropathy. *Muscle Nerve.* 2007;36:411–423.

Kincaid J. Neuropathies due to amyloidosis. In: Donofrio P, ed. *Textbook of Peripheral Neuropathy* (pp. 227–232). New York: Demos Medical; 2012.

Cancer-Related Polyneuropathies

John C. Kincaid MD

Description

Neuropathies in the form of neuronopathy, multiple mononeuropathy, or a generalized polyneuropathy can occur in patients who have cancer.

Neuropathy related to the treatment of cancer is covered in Chapter 36 on medication-related neuropathy.

Etiology

- Indirect (remote) effect due to autoimmune attack against peripheral neurons
- Direct effect due to neoplastic cell infiltration of peripheral nerves
- Indirect effect due to alteration of systemic and nerve metabolism

Epidemiology

Neuropathy is clinically evident in up to 5% of cancer patients but may be present in up to 30% of patients who are evaluated by nerve conduction study and quantitative sensory testing.

Pathogenesis

Syndrome 1: Sensory neuronopathy

- The most classic cancer-related neuropathy, but is very rare
- An autoimmune attack against the Hu protein complex present on certain neoplastic cells and sensory neurons is the presumed cause of this "paraneoplastic" or "remote effect of cancer" syndrome
- Small cell lung cancer is the most common neoplasm producing this syndrome, but breast, ovarian, and renal cancers also have been associated

Syndrome 2: Multiple mononeuropathy, plexopathy, or polyradiculopathy

- Infiltration of the nerve roots, brachial or lumbosacral plexi, or individual nerve trunks by neoplastic cells is the cause of this syndrome
- Leukemia or lymphoma is the more common source of infiltrating cells
- Cranial nerve syndromes are most often related to nasopharyngeal cancers
- Brachial plexopathy is most often associated with breast or lung cancers
- Lumbosacral plexopathy is most often associated with colon or cervical cancers

Syndrome 3: Generalized sensory-motor polyneuropathy

- Occurs in patients who have cancer but have not yet received chemotherapy or for which another etiology is definable

Risk Factors

Having cancer: especially small cell lung, breast, colon, nasopharyngeal, or leukemia

Clinical Features

- Syndrome 1: Abrupt to subacute onset of progressive sensory loss in the limbs and at times truncal areas producing impairment of standing and walking due to ataxia which may allow spontaneous movements of the hands or feet to develop (pseudoathetosis)
  - Some patients with this syndrome may also develop an encephalopathy with features of memory loss and seizures
- Syndrome 2: Abrupt to subacute onset of progressive focal pain, sensory, and motor dysfunction in single or multiple adjacent peripheral nerves or plexus territories
- Syndrome 3: Subacute onset of distal sensory and motor dysfunction in patients known to have or who are found to have cancer but who have not yet received chemotherapy or radiation therapy

Natural History

- Syndrome 1: Progressive worsening over weeks to a few months
- Syndrome 2: Progressive worsening producing more extensive focal deficits in the area of initial involvement
- Syndrome 3: Initial worsening and then stabilization

Diagnosis

Differential diagnosis

- Polyneuropathies due to concomitant conditions such as diabetes
- Chemotherapy-induced peripheral neuropathy
- Guillain-Barré syndrome or chronic inflammatory neuropathy
- Spinal cord or brain lesions due to metastases
- Local nerve lesions such as Herpes Zoster due to cancer-related immune system alteration

History

- Syndrome 1: Subacute onset of progressive sensory loss in the limbs resulting in impaired use of the hands and feet plus truncal ataxia
- Syndrome 2: Acute to subacute onset in individual or multiple cranial nerves or plexus dysfunction producing pain, sensory loss, and weakness in the affected nerve territories
- Syndrome 3: Subacute onset of length-dependent, sensory-motor dysfunction; alternatively, signs of peripheral neuropathy may be found on clinical examination and electrophysiologic testing without the patient being aware of the deficit

Physical examination

Syndrome 1

- Decreased sensation to vibration, light touch, position, and pain stimuli in the limbs and at times the truncal areas
- Absence or reduction of muscle stretch reflexes
- Muscle strength is normal but the sensory loss may be profound enough that the patient has to look directly at the body part being tested to be able to generate normal power
- Spontaneous movements of the toes, fingers, feet, hands, and at times truncal areas of which the patient may be unaware (pseudoathetosis) can occur when the sensory impairment is severe

Syndrome 2

- Focal sensory and motor deficits corresponding to individual or multiple adjacent cranial nerves or to the brachial or lumbosacral plexus

Syndrome 3

- Distal sensory loss to all modalities
- Weakness of toe, foot, and finger motions
- Loss of muscle stretch reflexes distally

Testing

- Anti-Hu antigen in serum and cerebrospinal fluid for syndrome 1
- Cerebrospinal fluid analysis for low glucose level and presence of neoplastic cells in syndrome 2

- Electrodiagnostic testing
  - Syndrome 1 shows absence of sensory nerve responses but normal values for motor studies
  - Syndrome 2 shows motor and sensory as well as needle EMG abnormalities in the areas of abnormality but may not show generalized abnormality
  - Syndrome 3 shows a distal predominant axonal-type peripheral neuropathy
- Imaging studies to define local abnormalities in cranial nerve, skull base, plexus, or multiple nerve root territories
- Standard serum tests for peripheral neuropathy: fasting glucose, vitamin B12 level, serum protein electrophoresis for monoclonal gammopathy

Treatment

- Syndrome 1: Management of the neoplasm is the mainstay, immunologically based treatments such as plasmapheresis or intravenous immune globulin probably do not improve the neuropathy
- Syndrome 2: Local radiation therapy and intrathecal chemotherapy
- Syndrome 3: Symptomatic management of sensory and motor deficits

Prognosis

- Syndrome 1: Defined by the course of primary neoplasm but sensory deficits tend to not improve
- Syndrome 2: Defined by the course of the primary neoplasm, but local deficits may improve temporarily with focused treatment
- Syndrome 3: Stable to slowly worsening course

Suggested Readings

Amato A, Russell J. *Neuromuscular Disorders* (pp. 313–332). New York: McGraw Hill; 2008.

Bosch P, Haberman T, Tefferi A. Peripheral neuropathy associated with lymphoma, leukemia and myeloprolif-erative disorders. In: Dyck PJ, Thomas PK, eds. *Peripheral Neuropathy*. 4th ed. (pp. 2489–2503). Philadelphia, PA: Elsevier; 2005.

II: Polyneuropathies

Chronic Inflammatory Demyelinating Polyradiculoneuropathy

John C. Kincaid MD

Description

Acquired, autoimmune sensory and motor polyneuropathy, which reaches maximum clinical deficit over a time course of at least 8 weeks, often evolving over a many-month course of time

Etiology

Autoimmune process, which attacks the myelin sheath and axons of the nerve roots and peripheral nerve trunks

Epidemiology

Prevalence of one case per 100,000 population

Pathogenesis

- Cellular rather than antibody-mediated autoimmune response, which cross reacts with antigens on the peripheral myelin sheath or axons of the nerve roots and nerve trunks
- Immunoglobulin M (IgM) monoclonal gammopathy with cross reaction against the myelin-associated glycoprotein component of peripheral nerve may produce this syndrome

Risk Factors

- IgM monoclonal gammopathy
- Antecedent events such as infectious illnesses before the onset of neuropathy are much less common, in contrast to the situation for Guillain-Barré syndrome

Clinical Features

- "Ascending" (distal to proximal, lower extremity somewhat earlier than upper extremity) pattern of motor and sensory deficits, with motor dysfunction usually being the more prominent feature
- Maximum deficit is reached in a time course of more than 8 weeks; a time frame of many months to few years is more typical
- Loss of muscle stretch reflexes
- Neuropathic pain is usually not a prominent feature
- Autonomic dysfunction manifesting as unstable blood pressure or cardiac arrhythmias may occur
- Urinary function is disturbed in approximately 25% of patients

Natural History

- Spontaneous improvement is uncommon
- A relapsing remitting course occurs in about 50% of patients

Diagnosis

Differential diagnosis

- Subacutely evolving polyneuropathy due to diabetes, alcoholism, amyloidosis, HIV infection, autoimmune conditions such as Sjögren syndrome or systemic lupus erythematosus, and inherited neuropathies
- Spinal cord compression due to cervical or lumbosacral spondylotic myelopathy
- Residual of prior lesions such as polio and post-polio syndrome

History

- Paresthesias begin in the feet and spread proximally into the legs and upper extremities in a time course extending over at least 8 weeks but more typically over many months
- Weakness, which evolves in the same distal to proximal, lower, and upper extremity pattern described in clinical features
- Neuropathic pain is not usually a prominent feature

Physical examination

- Symmetric weakness in distal and proximal muscles of the lower and upper extremities
- Weakness of facial muscles occurs in 15% of patients and tends to be mild
- Papilledema can occur when cerebrospinal fluid protein is very high
- Respiratory insufficiency is unusual in this condition
- Loss of muscle stretch reflexes
- Deficits in sensory functions such as light touch, vibration, and pin prick sensation

Testing

- Motor nerve conduction studies show prolongation of distal latencies and slowing of conduction velocities in forearm and leg segments of the nerves.
- Distal latencies >125% of the upper limit of normal, conduction velocities <70% of the low limit of normal

and conduction block with response amplitudes dropping by more than 20% between proximal and distal stimulus sites support the neuropathy being predominantly demyelinating

- Sensory conduction studies also become abnormal by showing prolonged distal latencies and reduction of response amplitudes, but nerves that do not pass through potential entrapment sites such as the sural and superficial radial may remain normal.
- The latencies of the F-wave and H-reflex become prolonged if they are recordable
- Needle EMG shows reduction of motor unit potential recruitment as the weakness begins and then may show fibrillations and positive waves by 4 to 8 weeks after onset, reflecting the development of axonal dysfunction
- Cerebrospinal fluid (CSF) protein is elevated by cell count remains normal
- Porphyria screen, vitamin B12 level, serum protein electrophoresis for monoclonal protein, especially IgM

Treatment

- Immune-modulating therapy with corticosteroids, plasma exchange, or intravenous infusion of gamma-globulin should produce improvement in 80% of patients
- Ongoing treatment over months to years may be required

Prognosis

- Spontaneous improvement is rare
- Immune-modulating treatment should produce improvement in up to 80% of patients but prolonged treatment may be required

Suggested Readings

Amato A, Russell J. *Neuromuscular Disorders* (pp. 233–260). New York: McGraw Hill; 2008.

Hahn A, Hartung H, Dyck P. Chronic inflammatory demyelinating polyradiculoneuropathy. In: Dyck PJ, Thomas PK, eds. *Peripheral Neuropathy.* 4th ed. (pp. 2221–2253). Philadelphia, PA: Elsevier; 2005.

II: Polyneuropathies

Critical Illness Polyneuropathy

Gentry Dodd MD ■ John C. Kincaid MD

Description

An acute, acquired, axonal polyneuropathy that develops during the treatment of some severely ill patients

Etiology

- Occurs in conditions such as sepsis, severe trauma, or pancreatitis, which provoke the systemic inflammatory response syndrome (SIRS)

Epidemiology

- Fifty-eight percent of patients with a prolonged intensive care unit (ICU) stay develop critical illness neuropathy
- It has been found in some prospective studies that 70% to 80% of patients with severe sepsis and multiple organ failure suffer from this disorder
  - It is seen in nearly 100% of patients with sepsis and coma
- Patients who end up developing critical illness neuropathy have an increased organ dysfunction score and a number of organs involved and are also ventilated longer

Pathogenesis

Proposed mechanisms include effects of inflammatory mediators such as cytokines, interleukins, and alteration of nitric oxide pathway functioning

Risk Factors

Sepsis, severe trauma, and conditions such as pancreatitis, which result in the patient being ill enough to require mechanical ventilation

Clinical Features

- Onset while the patient is in intensive care
- Inability to wean from mechanical ventilation is usually the most prominent manifestation
- Weakness in a distal to proximal gradient but which can be severe enough to produce complete limb and respiratory muscle paralysis
- Loss of reflexes while in ICU
- Abnormal sensation in a distal to proximal gradient (this feature may not be apparent if the patient has an altered sensorium)
- Neuropathic pain in the limbs may occur but is usually not a prominent feature

- Autonomic dysfunction is not a major feature or is not clearly distinguishable from the effects of the primary illness
- Urinary and rectal sphincter functions usually remain normal

Natural History

Improves over 3 to 12 months in most patients who are able to be discharged from the hospital.

Diagnosis

Differential diagnosis

- Critical illness myopathy
- Acute polyneuropathy due to other causes such as Guillain-Barré Syndrome, cancer chemotherapy, nitrofurantoin exposure, or porphyria
- Cervical spinal cord lesion due to an inflammatory process such as transverse myelitis or the initial attack of multiple sclerosis
- Spinal cord infarction
- Botulism

History

- Weakness of the limbs and truncal muscles, which develops while the patient is in ICU and most often manifests as difficulty weaning the patient from the ventilator
- Dysesthesias in feet and hands with onset in the same time frame as the motor deficits but which may not be apparent due to altered sensorium and impaired communication due to intubation

Physical examination

- Symmetrical weakness of the lower and upper extremities affecting both distal and proximal muscles and often to the degree of producing complete paralysis of the limbs
- Respiratory failure due to pharyngeal, diaphragmatic, or chest wall muscle weakness occurs in 30% of patients
- Loss of muscle stretch reflexes
- Deficits in sensory function such as light touch, vibration, and pin prick sensation if the patient's sensorium allows reliable examination

Testing

- Conduction studies show an "axonal" pattern of abnormality: motor and sensory response amplitudes are low if present, conduction velocities are no slower than the mid-30 meters per second range, and distal latencies remain normal
- Needle EMG shows fibrillations and positive waves along with severely reduced motor unit potential recruitment
- Cerebrospinal fluid values tend to be normal
- Spinal cord magnetic resonance imaging (MRI) does not show significant abnormalities of the canal or spinal cord parenchyma
- Creatine phosphokinase values may be elevated early in the course of the weakness

Pitfalls

- In some patients that present similarly to those with critical illness neuropathy, may demonstrate reduced compound muscle action potentials with normal sensory amplitudes. In these cases, myopathies and disorders of neuromuscular transmission need to be considered
  - This can be done with creatine phosphokinase levels, muscle biopsy, and repetitive stimulation studies

Red flags

- Administration of succinylcholine as a muscle relaxing anesthetic agent runs the risk of hyperkalemic cardiac arrest

Treatment

Medical treatment

- Prevention of SIRS is the most effective way to reduce the chance of developing critical illness neuropathy
- Once critical illness neuropathy has been established, the only effective treatment is physical and occupational therapy
- The occurrence of critical illness neuropathy, however, has been shown to be reduced with intensive insulin treatment
  - Goal blood glucose level is 108–150 mg/dL
  - This should only be implemented by an experienced team

Exercise

- Once the patient is out of the ICU and able to tolerate therapy, focus should be on preserving the residual strength as well as preventing any type of contractures from forming

- There is a paucity of evidence suggesting that early rehabilitation beginning in the ICU enhances muscle recovery:
  - Early physical therapy (PT) and occupational therapy (OT) have been shown to improve functional independence
  - Range-of-motion exercises during bed rest should be established in ICU patients

Modalities

- Functional electrical stimulation
- Electrical stimulation (E stim)

Consults

- Physical and occupational therapy
- Neurology
- Physiatry

Complications of treatment

- Hypoglycemic events are significantly increased with the use of intensive insulin therapy
- Those patients receiving intensive insulin therapy have been shown to have a small increase in mortality

Prognosis

- In a study from 1996, a third of patients died in the acute phase, a third were ambulatory within 4 months, and the rest took 4 to 12 months to recover or remained ventilated
- Many patients have profound muscle weakness and chronic disability
- Persistent disabilities often include reduced reflexes, sensory loss, atrophic muscles, painful dysesthesias, and foot drop

Helpful Hint

- Examination of patients with possible critical illness polyneuropathy is often difficult to perform, given that the patient may be unresponsive, encephalopathic, or sedated.

Suggested Readings

Bolton C, Gilbert J, Hahn A. Polyneuropathy in critically ill patients. *J Neurol Neurosurg Psychiatry.* 1984;47:1223.

Zochodne D. Neuropathies associated with renal failure, hepatic disorders, chronic respiratory disease and critical Illness. In: Dyck PJ, Thomas PK, eds. *Peripheral Neuropathy.* 4th ed. (pp. 2017–2037). Philadelphia, PA: Elsevier; 2005.

Hereditary Motor and Sensory Neuropathy/Charcot-Marie-Tooth Disease

John C. Kincaid MD

Description
Inherited polyneuropathy, which most often causes motor dysfunction more prominently than sensory dysfunction

Etiology
Genetically based alteration of structural components of the Schwann cell, axon, or neuronal cell body of peripheral neurons

Epidemiology
- Prevalence of one case per 100,000 population
- Dominant inheritance is the most common genetic pattern but X-linked and recessive patterns also occur

Pathogenesis
- Charcot-Marie-Tooth (CMT) patients usually segregate into demyelinating (CMT type 1) or axonal (CMT type 2) forms depending on the degree of nerve conduction velocity slowing
- Alerted structure in a growing list of proteins involved in Schwann cell or axon function of peripheral neurons is the basis of the clinical manifestation
- Abnormalities of Schwann cell proteins, such as peripheral membrane protein 22 (PMP-22) and myelin protein zero (MPZ), are the more commonly identified alterations in the demyelinating form of the disease
- Abnormalities in a mitochondrial cell wall protein (mitofusion-2) is the most common alteration found in CMT type 2 patients
- Abnormalities in a gap junction protein present in Schwann cell membranes (connexin 32) accounts for most of the X-linked varieties of CMT

Risk Factors
- A parent having the same condition: dominant inheritance is the most common, but X-linked and recessive patterns also occur

Clinical Features
- Gradual onset, most often in the late teen age-group, of a pattern of weakness involving the toes and feet initially and then the fingers/hands years later
- Abnormalities in sensory function tend to be a less prominent symptom, despite sensory deficits being present on clinical examination
- Neuropathic pain tends to not be a prominent feature in most patients
- Reflexes are abnormal distally but may be preserved proximally
- Except for distal limb abnormalities in sweating, autonomic functions tend to be clinically spared
- Urinary and rectal sphincter functions usually remain normal
- A pattern of recurrent mononeuropathies, such as foot drop, wrist drop, or ulnar deficits, which come on after prolonged position maintenance and then improve over weeks to months, can be seen in the hereditary liability to pressure palsy variant of CMT type 1

Natural History
Gradual onset over years, most often in the late teens or early twenties, with very slow worsening over subsequent years to decades

Diagnosis

Differential diagnosis
- Other slowly evolving neuropathies such as those due to diabetes or excessive alcoholic consumption
- Late-onset, lower motor neuron disorders such as spinal muscular atrophy
- Spinocerebellar ataxias

History
- Weakness in toe and ankle functions, which begins insidiously, manifesting as foot drop followed years later by onset of finger and hand weakness
- Distal sensory symptoms such as numbness and tingling, which appear in a similar time frame but which are often much less prominent than the motor manifestations

Physical examination
- Symmetrical weakness in distal muscles of the lower and, to a lesser degree, upper extremities

- Atrophy of intrinsic foot and distal leg muscles producing a "peroneal muscular atrophy" pattern (stork or inverted champagne bottle legs)
- Atrophy of intrinsic hand muscles, which becomes more prominent years after the foot weakness and atrophy
- Abnormal foot structure is often present from childhood: pes cavus, abnormally high-arched feet
- Loss of muscle stretch reflexes distally
- Deficits in sensory functions of light touch, vibration, and pin prick sensation
- Superficial nerve trunks may be visually or palpably enlarged in some forms of the illness

Testing

- Motor nerve conduction studies most often show "demyelinating"-type abnormalities with prolongation of distal latencies and slowing of conduction velocities in leg and forearm segments of the nerves
- Distal latencies > 125% of the upper limit of normal, conduction velocities < 70% of the lower limit of normal
- Axonal (CMT type 2) varieties show reduction in response amplitudes but only mild slowing of conduction velocities
- Conduction block tends to not be found unless the patient has hereditary liability to pressure palsy variant of neuropathy
- Sensory conduction studies also become abnormal by showing prolonged distal latencies and reduction of response amplitudes

- The latencies of the F-wave and H-reflex become prolonged if they are recordable
- Needle EMG shows fibrillations, positive waves, and enlarged motor unit potentials in patients who have been symptomatic for years or decades
- Genetic testing for the commonly identified protein abnormalities such as PMP-22, MPZ, and connexin 32

Treatment

- No direct treatment currently exists
- Ankle foot orthoses can improve stability in standing and walking
- Physical and occupation therapy to maximize capabilities
- Antineuropathic pain medications if paresthesias and neuropathic pain are significant symptoms

Prognosis

- Slow worsening over decades
- Progression to a wheel chair–dependent state is uncommon

Suggested Readings

Amato A, Russell J. *Neuromuscular Disorders.* (pp 162–192). New York: McGraw Hill; 2008.

Griffin J, Sheikh K. The Guillain-Barré Syndromes. In: Dyck PJ, Thomas PK, eds. *Peripheral Neuropathy.* 4th ed. (pp 2197–2219). Philadelphia, PA: Elsevier; 2005.

II: Polyneuropathies

Idiopathic Polyneuropathy

John C. Kincaid MD

Description
Sensory-motor polyneuropathy occurring in patients for whom an etiology has not been determined

Etiology
No etiology has been established despite an adequate workup.

Epidemiology
About 30% of adults who develop polyneuropathy will not have an etiology established.

Pathogenesis
An axonal-type mechanism is presumed based on the characteristics of nerve conduction studies in this group of patients

Clinical Features
- Insidious onset and slow progression is the most common pattern
- A length-dependent sensory or sensory-motor pattern is expected
- Reflex loss should be consistent with the clinical deficits rather than being generalized when other clinical deficits are still mild
- Foot deformities such as hammer toes and pes cavus should not be present
- Some patients will have a "small fiber neuropathy" pattern with abnormalities in pain and thermal sensory modalities only

Natural History
Onset over months to years with very slow progression over the following years is the most common pattern

Diagnosis

Differential diagnosis
- Polyneuropathy related to glucose intolerance
- Chronic inflammatory polyneuropathy
- Cervical or lumbar canal stenosis
- Medication, toxin, or infection-related neuropathy
- Neuropathy due to monoclonal gammopathy
- Neuropathy due to inflammatory connective tissue diseases such as Sjögren's syndrome
- Genetic neuropathy when details of family history are limited
- Postgastric bypass-related neuropathy
- Prior therapeutic radiation treatment

History
- Slow onset of numbness, paresthesias, and, at times, burning pain in the toes and feet
- Significant distal weakness or ataxia are usually not features of this type of neuropathy

Physical examination
- Deficits in distal lower extremities in sensory modalities of light touch, vibration, pin prick, and hot and cold sensation
- Mild symmetrical weakness of foot and distal lower extremity muscles may be present
- Loss of muscle stretch reflexes proportionate to the other clinical deficits
- Toe and foot deformities suggestive of an inherited etiology should be absent

Testing
- Biochemical and serological assessment, including fasting glucose, renal function, hematologic status, vitamin B12 level, serum and urine protein electrophoresis, connective tissue diseases, HIV, and hepatitis B and C
- Glucose tolerance testing should be considered if an etiology remains unestablished
- Cerebrospinal fluid analysis will likely not be helpful and will be normal or show nonspecific abnormalities such as mild elevation of protein
- Conduction studies will usually show an "axonal" pattern of abnormality: motor and sensory response amplitudes are reduced if present, conduction velocities are no slower than the mid-30 meters per second range and distal latencies remain normal
- Needle EMG shows fibrillations and positive waves in foot and distal leg muscles along with abnormally large motor unit potentials in distal muscles

- Spinal cord magnetic resonance imaging (MRIs) do not show significant abnormalities of the neural foramina, spinal canal dimensions, or the spinal cord parenchyma.
- Genetic screening and assessment for the presence of antinerve antibodies should not be done unless the clinical scenario is suggestive of an etiology in these categories.
- Nerve biopsy will usually not be helpful in establishing a specific diagnosis
- Skin biopsy for quantitation of intraepidermal nerve fiber density should be considered if a "small fiber" neuropathy pattern is present and the evaluation has not revealed a specific cause.

Treatment

- Symptomatic treatment of paresthesias and neuropathic pain
- Continued neurological follow up

Prognosis

Most patients do not progress to significant levels of impairment

Suggested Readings

Amato A, Russell J. *Neuromuscular Disorders* (pp. 361–370). New York: McGraw Hill; 2008.

Hughes R, Umapathi T. A controlled investigation of the cause of chronic idiopathic axonal polyneuropathy. *Brain.* 2004;127: (pp. 1723–1730).

II: Polyneuropathies

Medication-Induced Polyneuropathy

John C. Kincaid MD

Description

Acquired polyneuropathies arising as side effects from medication usage

Etiology

Disruption of cellular functions involved in the maintenance of the axon and neuronal cell body

Epidemiology

Most often encountered in patients undergoing treatment for cancer, cardiac arrhythmia, subacute to chronic infections, and rheumatologic disorders

Pathogenesis

- Disruption of axoplasmic transport
- Interference with mitochondrial and nuclear DNA translation
- Other incompletely understood mechanisms

Risk Factors

- Exposure to any of the following medications, typically in a dose-related fashion: amiodarone, bortezomib, cis- or oxaliplantin, colchicine, cytosine arabinoside, dapsone, etopside, chloroquine or hydroxychloroquine, isoniazid, leflunomide, metronidazole, nitrofurantoin, nucleosides for HIV, paclitaxel, phenytoin, pyridoxine in excessive amounts, thalidomide and vincristine
- Pre-existing inherited or diabetic polyneuropathy may result in a more prominent neuropathy than attributable to medication exposure alone

Clinical Features

- Length-dependent sensory-motor polyneuropathy producing distal sensory loss, neuropathic pain, and weakness of toe and ankle musculature is the most common manifestation
- Sensory-only pattern of symptoms and signs such as paresthesia and ataxia may occur with medications such as the platinum-based chemotherapeutic drugs
- Subacute onset and progression related to cumulative dosing is the most common clinical pattern but acute onset can be seen, for example, nitrofurantoin exposure
- Autonomic dysfunction manifesting as impaired bowel motility and urinary retention may occur with vincristine

Natural History

- A pattern of subacute onset and progression, which then improves over months after exposure ends, is the most common syndrome
- The clinical pattern termed "coasting", in which manifestations continue to worsen for several weeks after the exposure ends, can also be seen

Diagnosis

Differential diagnosis

- Acute to subacute polyneuropathy due to other causes, such as Guillain-Barré, chronic inflammatory neuropathy, porphyria, or spread of the neoplasm to the cranial nerves or nerve roots
- Spinal cord lesion due to an inflammatory process such as transverse myelitis or the initial attack of multiple sclerosis
- Spinal cord compression due to spondylotic myelopathy or metastasis to the spinal column

History

- Numbness, paresthesias, and pain beginning in the toes and spreading proximally into the feet, legs, and upper extremities over weeks to months during exposure to the medication
- Weakness which evolves in a similar distal to proximal, lower and upper extremity pattern, to that described for sensory dysfunction

Physical examination

- Deficits in sensory function, such as light touch, vibration, pin prick and temperature sensations; more prominent distally
- Ataxia may be present if the sensory loss is severe
- Symmetrical weakness in distal muscles of the lower and then upper extremities
- Loss of muscle stretch reflexes in a length-dependent pattern
- Deficits in cranial nerve function are uncommon and their presence suggests alternative explanations such as spread of the neoplasm to the meninges

Testing

- Motor nerve conduction studies show reduced amplitudes of sensory and motor responses along with mild slowing of conduction velocities in lower and upper extremity nerves
- Distal latencies should remain normal and conduction block should not occur
- The latencies of the F-wave and H-reflex remain normal or are only slightly prolonged, as long as they are still recordable
- Needle EMG may show fibrillations and positive waves if motor axons are affected. Abnormally large motor unit potentials can occur months to years later as reinnervation occurs

Treatment

- Neuroprotective agents that lessen the tendency for development of the neuropathy do not yet exist

- Symptomatic management of the sensory disturbances
- Physical and occupational therapy if significant motor and coordination deficits develop
- Reassurance that the deficits will likely improve over months after the medication exposure ends

Prognosis

Improvement over months to about 2 years after exposure to the medication ends

Suggested Readings

Amato A, Russell J. *Neuromuscular Disorders* (pp. 323–349). New York: McGraw Hill; 2008.

Herskovitz S, Schaumburg H. Neuropathy caused by drugs. In: Dyck PJ, Thomas PK, eds. *Peripheral Neuropathy*. 4th ed. (pp. 2553–2583). Philadelphia, PA: Elsevier; 2005.

Multifocal Motor Neuropathy

John C. Kincaid MD

Description

Acquired, autoimmune polyneuropathy, which produces asymmetric dysfunction of multiple individual peripheral nerves (multifocal), with motor deficits usually being predominant over sensory

Etiology

- Autoimmune process producing focal dysfunction of the myelin sheath and axons of multiple individual peripheral nerve trunks
- Classified by some as a variant of chronic inflammatory polyneuropathy

Epidemiology

- Annual incidence is 10 times less common than amyotrophic lateral sclerosis
- Male-female ratio of 3:1
- Tends to occur in the adult age group

Pathogenesis

- Autoimmune response against antigens thought to be localized to the peripheral myelin of motor axons
- Humoral (antibody) mechanisms are thought to be the predominant mechanism, and serum immunoglobulin M (IgM) antibodies directed against the GM1 ganglioside component of the peripheral nerve are present in many patients with this syndrome

Risk Factors

None have been identified

Clinical Features

- Weakness, fasciculations, and cramping in multiple individual peripheral nerve territories
- Muscle atrophy is present in cases of longer duration
- Onset tends to be gradual and initially involves a single nerve only, for example, radial, musculocutaneous, or peroneal
- Spread to other nerves in the same or other limbs occurs over months to years but evolution to a symmetrical pattern of involvement is not typical
- Muscle stretch reflexes become abnormal in the affected nerves but tend to not become diffusely abnormal

- Sensory symptoms occur in some patients but tend to be much less prominent than the motor dysfunction (Lewis-Sumner syndrome)
- Neuropathic pain is usually not a prominent feature
- Autonomic dysfunction in a widespread fashion causing blood pressure, cardiac, or sphincter abnormalities does not occur

Natural History

- Spontaneous improvement is uncommon
- Spread to additional individual nerves occurs over a many-month to many-year time frame

Diagnosis

Differential diagnosis

- Amyotrophic lateral sclerosis, producing lower motor neuron dysfunction
- Mononeuritis multiplex due to vasculitis affecting the vasa nervorum
- Hereditary liability to pressure palsy due to genetic abnormality in peripheral membrane protein (PMP)-22

History

- Motor dysfunction in a focal pattern: unilateral foot drop, wrist drop, elbow flexion
- Onset of individual lesions is usually insidious
- Spread to additional nerves occurs over months
- Abrupt onset of paresthesias and neuropathic pain typical of vasculitic mononeuritis multiplex is not a prominent feature
- Symptoms and signs of sensory dysfunction occur in some patients but tend to be much less prominent than the motor abnormalities

Physical examination

- Focal weakness in multiple individual peripheral nerve territories
- Atrophy can occur but early in the course of the illness, weakness can be disproportionate to the degree of atrophy
- Fasciculations can occur in the muscles of the affected nerves
- Reflexes are reduced or absent in the affected nerves but generalized areflexia typical of chronic inflammatory demyelinating polyradiculoneuropathy does not usually occur

- Signs of upper motor neuron dysfunction, as would be expected in typical amyotrophic lateral sclerosis (ALS), are not present
- Deficits in light touch, vibration, and pin prick sensation may be found in the sensory territories of the affected nerves

Testing

- Motor nerve conduction studies show partial conduction block along the course of the affected nerves, often at sites other than standard entrapment sites such as the ulnar at the elbow, the median at the wrist, or peroneal at the fibular head
- Slowing of conduction velocity and prolongation of distal latency is often present in affected nerves, whereas adjacent nerves remain electrically normal
- Sensory conduction studies in the nerves showing motor abnormality can also become abnormal but are more often normal
- Needle EMG shows reduction of motor unit potential recruitment early on while deficits present for many months produce signs of axonal damage such as fibrillation potentials and abnormally large voluntary motor unit potentials
- Cerebrospinal fluid protein tends to remain normal
- Sedimentation rate tends to remain normal
- Antibodies associated with peripheral vasculitides such as polyarteritis nodosa or Wegener's granulomatosis should be absent
- S gM antibodies against the ganglioside GM1 or related components of peripheral myelin are present in 50% or more patients

- Prophyria screen, vitamin B12 level, serum protein electrophoresis for monoclonal protein, especially IgM and serum glucose should be normal

Treatment

- Immune-modulating therapy with intravenous infusion of gamma-globulin is the mainstay of treatment
- Ongoing treatment at monthly intervals for prolonged time frames may be required
- Corticosteroids and plasma exchange do produce improvement or stabilization of this condition
- Intravenous pulse cyclophosphamide may cause improvement of the deficits
- The role of additional agents such as rituximab in the long-term management of this condition remain to be established
- Physical and occupational therapy to aid improvement of function

Prognosis

- Spontaneous improvement is rare
- Immune-modulating treatment should produce at least some improvement in up to 80% of patients, but prolonged treatment may be required

Suggested Readings

Amato A, Russell J. *Neuromuscular Disorders* (pp. 233–260). New York: McGraw Hill; 2008.

Taylor B, Willison H. Multifocal motor neuropathy with conduction block. In: Dyck PJ, Thomas PK, eds. *Peripheral Neuropathy*. 4th ed. (pp. 2277–2298). Philadelphia, PA: Elsevier; 2005.

Neuropathy Due to Herpes Zoster (Shingles)

John C. Kincaid MD

Description
Mononeuropathies and radiculopathies due to infection with Herpes Zoster virus

Etiology
Localized inflammatory process in sensory ganglion cells and their peripheral axons resulting from reactivation of latent Herpes Zoster virus infection

Epidemiology
- Occurs in patients who had prior infection with Herpes Zoster (Varicella or Chicken Pox)
- Decades after the initial Varicella attack, reactivation of virus latent in sensory ganglia produces the attack of Herpes Zoster
- Attacks are 2 to 3 times more likely in otherwise normal patients older than 60 years
- Attacks are more common in patients who have hematologic neoplasms or who are immunocompromised

Pathogenesis
- Initial infection with Herpes Zoster occurs in childhood as Chicken Pox (Varicella)
- After resolution of the Chicken Pox, the virus persists as a latent infection in the sensory neurons of cranial and spinal nerves
- The virus can reactivate when cell-mediated immunity becomes compromised by age, physiological stress, cancer, autoimmune disease, or therapeutic immune suppression

Risk Factors
- Age over 60 years
- Compromise of normal immune function by underlying disease or immune suppressive treatment

Clinical Features
- Dermatomal pain lasting 4 to 6 weeks
- Vesicular skin rash in the affected dermatome appearing days to about 2 weeks after onset of the pain
- Most often only one cranial nerve sensory territory or one spinal dermatome is unilaterally affected, the 5th cranial and any of the thoracic levels being the more common sites
- Weakness in the associated myotome may be present in up to 30% of patients
- Up to 40% patients over 60 years may have persisting pain after the rash resolves: postherpetic neuralgia
- Lesions in the 5th cranial territory may be associated with a cerebral vasculitis, producing a stroke syndrome
- Lesions of the 7th nerve can produce Ramsay-Hunt syndrome: facial palsy and Herpetic rash in the external ear canal
- Development of the typical pattern of pain without appearance of the rash is possible: Zoster sine Herpete

Natural History
The dermatomal pain and skin rash resolve over about 4 to 6 weeks but patients older than 60 years may be left with pain, which does not improve.

Diagnosis

Differential diagnosis
- Cervical, thoracic, or lumbar radiculopathy due to disk herniation
- Idiopathic or postviral 7th nerve palsy
- Trigeminal neuralgia
- Diabetic truncal neuropathy
- Carcinomatous meningitis producing cranial and spinal nerve root lesions
- Genital Herpes outbreak if the pain and cutaneous lesion occurs in the perineal area

History
- Abrupt, unprovoked onset of persistent pain in a cranial nerve or spinal nerve root pattern
- Vesicular rash in the area of pain appearing days to a week after pain onset
- Localized weakness may occur in muscles supplied by the affected nerve, including the abdominal wall

Physical examination

- Unilateral vesicular rash corresponding to the sensory territory of the affected cranial or spinal nerve: up to three adjacent dermatomes may be affected
- Weakness in myotome of the affected nerve

Testing

- The diagnosis is usually able to be established by the history and examination
- Brain and spinal magnetic resonance imaging (MRI) to evaluate for alternative causes of the clinical deficits
- Sensory and at times motor nerve conduction studies and needle EMG will be abnormal in the affected nerves, if those are accessible for testing

Treatment

Antiviral treatment may shorten the intensity and duration of the attack:

- Acyclovir 800 mg orally five times daily for 7 days
- Valacyclovir 1000 mg orally three times daily or famciclovir 500 mg three times daily for one week are alternative treatments but are about six times as expensive as acyclovir

- Oral steroids along with the antiviral agents may lessen the tendency to develop postherpetic neuralgia but the literature in support for this is not strong.
- The pain of the initial attack and of postherpetic neuralgia may improve with antineuropathic pain medications such as gabapentin, pregabalin, amitriptyline, analgesics, and topical lidocaine patches.

Prognosis

- In most patients, the pain and rash resolves within 2 months
- Those with pain persisting beyond approximately 2 months will have persisting pain and sensory disturbances in the territory of the affected nerve

Suggested Readings

Glidden D, Tyler K. Herpes virus infection and peripheral neuropathy. In: Dyck PJ, Thomas PK, eds. *Peripheral Neuropathy*. 4th ed. (pp. 2117–2127). Philadelphia, PA: Elsevier; 2005.

Hirsch M. Herpes virus infections. In: Nabel E, ed. *ACP Medicine* [Section 7, Ch XXVI]. Hamilton, ON, Canada: Decker; 2013.

Neuropathy Due to Leprosy

John C. Kincaid MD

Description
Peripheral neuropathy syndromes occurring in patients who have leprosy

Etiology
Infection with *Mycobacterium leprae*

Epidemiology
- Rare syndrome in the United States, Canada, and Europe. Approximately 100 new cases per year in the United States, which occur in immigrants from endemic areas such as India, Brazil, Nepal, and Mozambique

Pathogenesis
- The bacterium infects the skin and then spreads to the Schwann cells of the peripheral nerves and produces deficits, most often in cooler body areas such as the ear lobes, elbows, knees, and lateral shins
- Resulting local inflammation may cause segmental enlargement of the nerves, whereas demyelination of nerves further enhances sensory deficits

Risk Factors
- Exposure to the bacterium, most often through nasal secretions of infected patients and less often via skin-to-skin contact
- Patients who develop leprosy are thought to have a genetically based deficit in cell-mediated immunity

Clinical Features
- Leprosy occurs in three forms: **Tuberculoid** in which skin lesions are present but infrequent, **Lepromatous** in which skin lesions are widespread, and **Borderline Lepromatous**, which falls in between
- In each of these forms, discrete areas of hypopigmented, anesthetic skin occur
- The paucity or abundance of the lesions defines the type of leprosy
- Motor deficits may occur when the main nerve trunks are involved
- Local anesthesia secondary to the nerve involvement can allow trauma to the toes and fingers to be undetected and result in mutilation of the affected areas

Natural History
- Stabilization of the number of individual lesions may occur in the Tuberculoid variety of the disease, but progression occurs in the Lepromatous form

Diagnosis

Differential diagnosis
Multiple mononeuropathy due to other causes, such as diabetes, vasculitis, inherited liability to pressure palsy, neurofibromatosis, and Wartenburg's sensory neuritis

History
- Insidious onset of patchy skin lesions, which produce sensory loss within the area of involvement
- Individual lesions may progress to involvement of individual territories such as the ulnar peroneal, greater auricular
- Neuropathic pain is not a feature and would be expected in lesions due to vasculitis

Physical examination
- Patchy, multifocal skin lesions with raised, erythematous borders and hypopigmented centers
- Loss of sensation in the center of these lesions
- Larger areas of sensory loss and motor deficit can occur corresponding to individual nerve trunks
- Nerves may become visually or palpably enlarged
- A multiple mononeuropathy or polyneuropathy pattern of involvement can occur in advanced infection characteristic of the Lepromatous form of the disease.

Testing
- Skin biopsy of lesions in the Tuberculoid form shows granuloma formation, presence of helper T cells and few bacilli
- Skin biopsy of lesions in the Lepromatous form shows the absence of granuloma formation, absence of helper T cells but the presence of suppressor T cells and abundant bacilli
- When an individual nerve trunk is clearly abnormal, biopsy shows inflammation and the presence of bacilli

- Nerve conduction studies show reduction of sensory and motor response amplitudes in individual peripheral nerves

Treatment

- Tuberculoid form: rifampin 600 mg once per month and dapsone 100 mg daily for 6 months
- Lepromatous and borderline Lepromatous forms: rifampin 600 mg once per month, clofazimine 300 mg once per month, and dapsone 100 mg daily for 12 months
- Insensate areas such as finger, toes, and feet, may require protective splinting

Prognosis

- Stabilization of the pattern of involvement but deficits may persist long term

Suggested Readings

Leonard M, Blumberg H. Infections due to *Mycobacterium leprae* and nontuberculous mycobacteria. In: Nabel E, ed. *ACP Medicine.* (Section 7, Chapter XXXIX). Hamilton, ON, Canada: Decker; 2013.

Sabin T, Swift T, Jacobson R. Neuropathy associated with leprosy. In: Dyck PJ, Thomas PK, eds. *Peripheral Neuropathy.* 4th ed. (pp. 2081–2108). Philadelphia, PA: Elsevier; 2005.

II: Polyneuropathies

Polyneuropathy Due to Chemical Toxins and Metals

John C. Kincaid MD

Description

Polyneuropathy due to exposure to hexacarbons, arsenic, lead, and thallium (also see the chapter on "Medication-Induced Polyneuropathy")

Etiology

Exposure to these chemical agents appears to disrupt cellular functions involved in maintenance of the axon

Schaumburg has suggested the following criteria to support the relationship of a suspected toxin to the neuropathy:

- A characteristic clinic picture should be present
- A definite and dose-related exposure should be present
- The neuropathy should be reproducible in experimental animals

Epidemiology

Polyneuropathy due to any of these agents is profoundly rare but knowledge of their clinical presentation and evaluation is important in differential diagnosis.

Pathogenesis

The mechanism of action of each of these agents is not well established for the nervous system or other organ manifestations.

Risk Factors

- Exposure to hexacarbons (*n*-hexane or methyl *n*-butyl ketone) occurs in either an industrial setting in which factory or workshop ventilation is inadequate or in a personal setting of sniffing (or huffing) glue, gasoline, hair spray, brake cleaner, or other similar products
- Exposure to arsenic and thallium most often currently occur in the setting of attempted suicide or homicide
- Exposure to lead occurs in battery and other lead-containing product manufacturing, lead smelting, and perhaps lead ammunition remaining in the body after a gun shot

Clinical Features

For lead-related neuropathy:

- Abdominal pain with constipation
- Motor deficits, beginning in finger extensors then wrist extensors and then intrinsic hand muscles; lower extremity deficits manifest later
- Sensory deficits are not prominent or do not occur

For arsenic- and thallium-related neuropathy:

- Acute gastrointestinal illness followed several days to a week later by onset of distal lower and upper extremity paresthesias followed by distal weakness
- Skin changes of sloughing and then hyperpigmentation of the palms and soles occur in arsenic toxicity
- Alopecia is a feature of thallium toxicity but may not be apparent for 2 to 3 weeks after exposure
- Mees' lines occur in the fingernails and toe nails with exposure to arsenic or thallium

For hexacarbon-related neuropathy:

- Gradual onset of numbness in the toes, feet, and fingers
- Distal weakness may appear with continued exposure

Natural History

- Long-term improvement occurs with elimination of exposure
- The clinical pattern of "coasting" in which manifestations continue to worsen for several weeks to about 4 months after the exposure ends can also be seen

Diagnosis

Differential diagnosis

- Acute polyneuropathy due to other causes, such as Guillain-Barré syndrome, medication reaction, porphyria
- Spinal cord lesion due to an inflammatory process such as transverse myelitis or the initial attack of multiple sclerosis

History

- Validating exposure to the agent may require investigation by the physician
- The historical details specific to each agent are given in the Clinical Features section

Physical examination

For neuropathy due to lead toxicity:

- Weakness of finger and wrist extensors, intrinsic hand muscles, and distal leg muscles
- Sensation tends to remain normal
- Mees' lines on fingernails and toenails

For the other agents:

- Deficits in sensory function such as light touch and vibration more so than pin prick and temperature sensations in the toes, feet, and fingers
- Symmetric weakness in distal muscles of the lower and then upper extremities
- Loss of muscle stretch reflexes in a length-dependent pattern
- Mees' lines, palmar hyperpigmentation, and alopecia in thallium toxicity

Testing

- Hemoglobin and hematocrit levels for anemia
- Red cell morphology for basophilic stippling in lead and arsenic toxicity
- Serum levels for lead: normal <40 μg/dL or <70 μg/dL for industrial workers
- Urine lead levels: normal <100 μg/dL in 24 hours or <300 μg/dL for industrial workers

- Urine arsenic levels: normal <25 μg/dL in 24 hours or <125 μg/dL for fish eaters
- Arsenic levels in hair or finger nails: <1 μg/g
- For all other than lead toxicity: motor nerve conduction studies show reduced amplitudes of sensory and motor responses along with mild slowing of conduction velocities in lower and upper extremity nerves
- Needle EMG may show fibrillations and positive waves and reduced motor unit potential recruitment in the acute setting

Treatment

- Elimination of exposure to the toxic agent
- The role of chelation therapy in patients with arsenic, lead, and thallium exposure is not fully established
- Symptomatic management of the sensory disturbances
- Physical and occupational therapy if significant motor and coordination deficits develop

Prognosis

Improvement over months after exposure to the causative agent ends.

Suggested Readings

Berger A, Schaumburg H. Neuropathy associated with industrial agents, metals and drugs. In: Dyck PJ, Thomas PK, eds. *Peripheral Neuropathy*. 4th ed. (pp. 2505–2525). Philadelphia, PA: Elsevier; 2005.

Windebank A. Metal neuropathy. In: Dyck PJ, Thomas PK, eds. *Peripheral Neuropathy*. 4th ed. (pp. 2527–2551). Philadelphia, PA: Elsevier; 2005.

Polyneuropathy Due to Nutritional Deficiency

John C. Kincaid MD

Description

Acquired polyneuropathy occurring in patients who develop deficiencies in vitamins or other metabolic factors essential for the maintenance of nerve structure and function

Etiology

Most often encountered in patients who have inadequate intake or inadequate absorption of the essential factor

Epidemiology

Occurs most often in alcoholism, prolonged vomiting, following gastric bypass for weight loss, or in very restrictive diets

Pathogenesis

- Deficiency of thiamine (B1), pyridoxine (B6), cobalamin (B12), alpha-tocopherol (E), or copper can alter the metabolism of peripheral and at times central axons
- Excessive intake of pyridoxine can also produce polyneuropathy

Risk Factors

- Extensive gastrointestinal surgery, including gastric bypass for weight loss
- Alcoholism
- Antitubercular treatment with isoniazid increases demand for pyridoxine
- Excessive use of pyridoxine can also produce polyneuropathy

Clinical Features

- Slow onset
- Sensory symptoms, which initially appear in the distal lower extremities and migrate proximally if the condition worsens
- Weakness in distal lower and at times upper extremity muscles
- Ataxia

Natural History

- Develops over months to years
- Does not improve without treatment

Diagnosis

Differential diagnosis

- Diabetic polyneuropathy
- Chronic inflammatory polyneuropathy
- Cervical or lumbar canal stenosis
- Idiopathic sensory-motor polyneuropathies

History

- Slow onset of numbness, paresthesias, and burning pain of the toes, feet, and at times fingers
- Unsteady balance
- Weakness of distal leg and at times finger muscles

Physical examination

- Distal lower and at times upper extremity deficits in sensory function, such as light touch, vibration, and pin prick sensation
- Loss of muscle stretch reflexes at the ankle
- Symmetric weakness of distal lower and, at times, distal upper extremity muscles
- Signs of upper motor neuron dysfunction may also be present in cobalamin and copper deficiency

Testing

- Conduction studies show an "axonal" pattern of abnormality: motor and sensory response amplitudes are reduced if present, conduction velocities are no slower than the mid-30 meters per second range, and distal latencies remain normal
- Needle EMG shows fibrillations and positive waves in foot and distal leg muscles along with abnormally large motor unit potentials in distal muscles
- Cerebrospinal fluid values tend to be normal
- Spinal cord magnetic resonance imaging (MRI) does not show significant abnormalities of the canal or spinal cord parenchyma
- Vitamin level testing

Treatment

- Dietary supplementation of the deficient element
- Reduction or elimination of alcohol intake
- Symptomatic treatment of paresthesias and neuropathic pain
- Symptomatic management of ataxia

Prognosis

- Some improvement over months to about 2 years

Suggested Readings

Amato A, Russell J. *Neuromuscular Disorders* (pp. 303–311). New York: McGraw Hill; 2008.

Saperstein D, Barohn R. Neuropathy associated with nutritional and vitamin deficiencies. In: Dyck PJ, Thomas PK, eds. *Peripheral Neuropathy.* 4th ed. (pp. 2051–2062). Philadelphia, PA: Elsevier; 2005.

Polyneuropathy Due to Vasculitis

John C. Kincaid MD

Description

Peripheral neuropathy syndrome occurring most often in a pattern of sequentially developing multiple mononeuropathies

Etiology

Autoimmune vasculitis affecting the vasa nervorum

Epidemiology

Rare syndrome approximately five cases per 100,000 population per year

Pathogenesis

- Vasculitis affecting arteries and capillaries, including those of the vasa nervorum, become involved due to an inflammatory response
- Other organ systems such as the sinuses, lungs, gastrointestinal tract, and kidneys may be involved concurrently, depending on the specific immune responses
- Infectious processes such as hepatitis B or C or HIV may trigger the vasculitis
- May occur as a component of systemic lupus erythematosus (SLE), rheumatoid arthritis (RA), Sjögren's syndrome or systemic sclerosis

Risk Factors

- Other autoimmune conditions such as SLE or RA
- Hepatitis B or C infections

Clinical Features

- Sensory disturbance with neuropathic pain and paresthesias occurring in a patchy, stepwise, progressive (multiple mononeuropathic) pattern over a many-week to several-month time frame
- Motor deficits that occur in the same stepwise pattern
- Evolution to a symmetric pattern of involvement may occur as additional individual nerves become involved
- Onset in a symmetrical pattern of involvement rather than the more typical progressive multi-focal one may also occur

Natural History

- Progressive worsening over weeks to months
- Spontaneous remission is not typical

Diagnosis

Differential diagnosis

- Other acute to subacute progressive polyneuropathies such as Guillain-Barré syndrome or chronic inflammatory neuropathy
- Multifocal motor neuropathy
- Hereditary liability to pressure palsy
- Brachial or lumbosacral plexopathy producing bilateral abnormality

History

- Abrupt onset of mononeuropathic-type sensory and motor deficits, which progress in a stepwise fashion to involve additional nerves in other limbs, the trunk and at times, the cranial region
- Neuropathic abnormalities most often occur as part of a syndrome involving other organ systems, such as the sinuses, lungs, gastrointenstinal tract, kidneys, joints, and skin, but the neuropathic manifestations may occur in isolation (nonsystemic vasculitic neuropathy)

Physical examination

- Patchy, multifocal deficits in motor and sensory function, which correspond to individual peripheral nerve territories
- Evidence of sinus, pulmonary, joint, and cutaneous involvement may be present, depending on the specific diagnosis

Testing

- Nerve conduction studies show reduction of sensory and motor response amplitudes in individual peripheral nerves with adjacent nerves initially remaining normal
- Conduction velocities in affected nerves tend to remain normal or be only mildly slowed in an "axonal" pattern of abnormality
- Needle EMG shows denervation in muscles of the affected nerves

- Test for elevation of sedimentation rate, presence of antineutrophil cytoplasmic antibodies (p or c), cryoglobulinemia, and antibodies or antigens for hepatitis B or C
- Assessment of sinuses, pulmonary, gastrointestinal, and renal systems to identify concurrent involvement
- Biopsy of a cutaneous nerve: sural, superficial peroneal, or radial, demonstrated to be abnormal by clinical examination or nerve conduction study to evaluate for presence of vasculitis
- Biopsy of muscle in an abnormal nerve territory may increase the yield for diagnosis of vasculitis

Treatment
- Immune modulation with corticosteroids, 1 mg/kg daily
- Concurrent use of a nonsteroidal agent such as cyclophosphamide given as monthly intravenous pulses improves the long-term course of the illness

- Symptomatic management of paresthesias and neuropathic pain by antiepileptic, antidepressant, and at times analgesic medications

Prognosis
- Stabilization of the pattern of involvement is the initial indication of responsiveness of the condition
- Improvement in the motor and sensory deficits over months is expected, but motor, sensory, and neuropathic pain deficits may persist long term

Suggested Readings
Amato A, Russell J. *Neuromuscular Disorders* (pp. 261–270). New York: McGraw Hill; 2008.
Collins M, Kissel J. Neuropathies with systemic vasculitis. In: Dyck PJ, Thomas PK, eds. *Peripheral Neuropathy*. 4th ed. (pp. 2335–2404). Philadelphia, PA: Elsevier; 2005.

Polyneuropathy in Diabetes Mellitus

John C. Kincaid MD

Description

Syndrome of symmetrical length-dependent polyneuropathy, which occurs in patients with diabetes mellitus or in "prediabetic" states

Etiology

Alteration in the microenvironment of the peripheral axons due to altered glucose metabolism

Epidemiology

- Produces symptoms in approximately 20% of diabetics with disease duration of over 10 years
- Is present in approximately 50% of that same population based on physical examination and neurophysiological assessment

Pathogenesis

- Accumulation of osmotically active sugars in the axons or Schwann cells (polyol pathway)
- Alteration of protein function by glycosylation
- Disturbance of microvascular functions in the peripheral nerves

Risk Factors

- Persistently poor control of serum glucose
- Metabolic syndrome
- Impaired glucose tolerance without frank hyperglycemia

Clinical Features

- Abnormal sensation in the toes, feet, distal legs, and fingers: numbness, tingling, pins, and needles in a symmetrical pattern
- Pain in the toes and feet (less common than the abnormal sensations listed earlier) with characteristics such as "deep in the bone" pressure, surface burning, short sharp jabs of knife-like pain
- Allodynia (painful sensation provoked by a nonpainful stimulus such as bed sheets), especially in the tips of the toes
- Ankle and hand weakness in more advanced cases

Natural History

- Slow worsening over years manifested by more proximal spread of the abnormal sensations
- Tight control of blood sugars lessens the tendency for progression in type 1 diabetes

Diagnosis

Differential diagnosis

- Plantar fascitis
- Tarsal tunnel syndrome (bilaterally)
- Interdigital neuroma (Morton's neuroma) bilaterally
- Other causes of polyneuropathy

History

- 25% to 30% may be asymptomatic and the neuropathy only be identified during physical examination or neurophysiological testing for another condition such as lumbar radiculopathy
- Numbness in the toes, which progresses proximally over years
- Pain and allodynia in the feet with or without other disturbances of sensation
- Asymmetric involvement of the lumbosacral plexus and/or the thoracic or upper lumbar truncal nerves may occur independent of the polyneuropathy (see the chapter on "Lumbosacral Plexopathy")
- Autonomic dysfunction as manifest by erectile dysfunction, impaired sweating in the distal limbs, orthostatic hypotension, and disturbed gastrointestinal motility

Physical examination

- Decreased sensation to vibratory, light touch, pin prick, or monofilament-type stimuli in toes and distal aspect of the feet
- Absence of ankle muscle stretch reflexes
- Weakness of toe abduction, flexion, or extension motions
- Weakness of ankle extension and flexion plus weakness of intrinsic hand muscles in more severe cases

Testing

- Nerve conduction studies show reduction of sensory response amplitudes in distal leg/foot nerves initially and then reduction of motor response amplitudes later. Conduction velocities become slowed but remain above 70% of the low limit of normal, and distal latencies tend to not be abnormally prolonged.

- Similar abnormalities may appear in hand nerves if the overall condition worsens over the years
- Abnormalities in autonomic control of the heart (cardiovagal) as demonstrated by heart rate with deep breathing testing

Treatment

- Optimal control of serum glucose
- Daily visual inspection of the soles
- Symptomatic management of paresthesias and neuropathic pain by antiepileptic, antidepressant, and at times analgesic medications

Prognosis

- Stable to slowly worsening symptoms and signs of the neuropathy
- Neuropathic pain, which begins after treatment of hyperglycemia begins, may improve over months if improved sugar control is maintained

Suggested Readings

Llewelyn J, Tomlinson D, Thomas P. Diabetic neuropathies. In: Dyck PJ, Thomas PK, eds. *Peripheral Neuropathy.* 4th ed. (pp. 2197–2219). Philadelphia, PA: Elsevier; 2005.

Rajabally Y. Neuropathy and impaired glucose tolerance: An updated review of evidence. *Acta Neurol Scand.* 2011;124:1–8.

II: Polyneuropathies

Polyneuropathy in Lyme Disease

John C. Kincaid MD

Description

Mononeuropathies and polyneuropathies due to infection with *Borrelia* (*B.*) *burgdorferi*.

The name Lyme is based on the features of the condition being characterized on a group of patients from the Lyme, Connecticut region.

Etiology

Inflammatory process due to either direct invasion of the affected nerves by the infectious agent or an immune response against the agent, which attacks the myelin and axons of peripheral nerve trunks or nerve roots.

Epidemiology

- Occurs in specific regions of North America and Europe: States of the New England area, Wisconsin, Minnesota, and Northern California
- May to August occurrence pattern

Pathogenesis

- Infection with *B. burgdorferi* and resulting humoral and cell-mediated immunological reaction to the agent
- The relative roles of direct invasion by the infectious agent versus immune responses against it in the pathogenesis of the neurologic lesions has not been fully established.

Risk Factors

- Living in or visiting an area of endemic infection during the late spring to early fall
- Being bitten by a tick—typically *Ixodes scapularis* (deer tick) or other *Ixodes* species—which carry *B. burgdorferi*

Clinical Features

- Red papular skin lesion (erythema migrans) appearing 7 to 10 days after the tick bite, which enlarges over days to a few weeks
- Low-grade fever, arthralgias, headache, and malaise may occur while the skin lesion is present
- 15% of patients develop signs of more clear cut neurologic involvement in the first 3 months after the tick bite: meningitis, cranial neuropathy, radiculitis
- 10% develop cardiac arrhythmia in the first few months of the illness

Natural History

The initial cutaneous and systemic manifestations improve, but the patient may develop longer-term effects such as arthritis, persistent fatigue, and encephalopathy.

Diagnosis

Differential diagnosis

- Idiopathic 7th nerve palsy
- Acute cervical, thoracic, or lumbar radiculopathy
- Viral meningitis
- Carcinomatous meningitis producing cranial and spinal nerve root lesions
- Autoimmune conditions producing multisystem symptoms and signs

History

- Development of an isolated skin lesion with features of erythema migrans in concert with experiencing a tick bite a few days to a few weeks previously
- Onset of unilateral or bilateral 7th nerve palsy, headache, or painful radiculopathy several weeks after appearance of the skin lesion
- Multijoint arthritis, especially in the knees, appearing several months after the skin lesion
- Late effects such as fatigue and cognitive impairment in a small percent of patients

Physical examination

- Red papular lesion appearing about 1 week after the tick bite, which enlarges over the next few days in a red ring border-clear center
- Unilateral or bilateral 7th nerve deficit
- Asymmetric "radicular" weakness and sensory loss with or without cranial nerve deficits
- Acute to subacute multijoint arthritis, especially in the knees

Testing

- Serology: Two-step testing of the antibody response against *B. burgdorferi* antigens (note: these may be negative in the first 2 weeks after onset)
  - Enzyme-linked immunosorbent assay (ELISA) or immunofluorscence assay (IFA) for IgM and IgG antibodies
  - If ELISA or IFA assay is positive, perform Western immunoblot test for antibodies
  - If both are positive, infection has occurred

- Cerebrospinal fluid testing may show pleocytosis but normal glucose levels
- Motor and sensory nerve conduction studies show an "axonal" pattern of abnormalities in the affected nerves

Treatment
- Patients with erythema migrans only: Oral amoxicillin 500 mg tid, doxycycline 100 mg bid or cefuroxime axetil 500 mg bid for 2 to 3 weeks with immune-modulating therapy by plasma exchange or intravenous infusion of gammaglobulin shortens the duration of the deficits by 30% to 50%
- Patients with facial palsy as a component of Lyme disease: Oral antibiotics as listed above for 30 days

- Patients with arthritis: Oral antibiotics as listed above for 2 months

Prognosis
- With appropriate antibiotic treatment, the majority of patients resolve the systemic, neurologic, and rheumatologic manifestations of the disease

Suggested Readings
Said G. Lyme disease. In: Dyck PJ, Thomas PK, eds. *Peripheral Neuropathy*. 4th ed. (pp. 2109–2116). Philadelphia, PA: Elsevier; 2005.

Tompkins D, Luft B. Lyme disease and other spirochetal zoonoses., In: Nabel E, ed. *ACP Medicine*. [Section 7, Chapter VII]. Hamilton, ON, Canada: Decker; 2013.

II: Polyneuropathies

Polyneuropathy Related to HIV Infection

John C. Kincaid MD

Description

Several syndromes of polyneuropathy or polyradiculopathy can occur in patients infected with HIV

Etiology

Infection with HIV and resulting alteration of immune-mediated responses, which then secondarily involve the peripheral nervous system

Epidemiology

20% to 30% of HIV-infected patients develop a clinically evident peripheral neuropathy related to the primary condition or the treatment thereof. A higher percentage of patients will be found to have neuropathy based on clinical and electrophysiological examinations rather than based on symptoms alone.

Pathogenesis

- The virus does not directly infect the peripheral nerves
- Syndrome 1: Immune response at the time of initial infection is likely the cause of the Guillain-Barré-type neuropathy, which can occur early in the course of the infection
- Syndrome 2: Immune response against the virus is the likely cause of the sensory-motor and often painful neuropathy encountered late in the course of HIV infection when AIDS develops
- Syndrome 3: Immune deficiency occurring in advanced stages of the illness allows opportunistic infections with cytomegalovirus (CMV) to develop and produce lumbosacral polyradiculitis

Risk Factors

- Infection with HIV virus
- Lack of adequate antiretroviral treatment

Clinical Features

- Syndrome 1: Abrupt to subacute onset of motor and sensory deficits in the lower and upper limbs is typical of Guillain-Barré syndrome, which occurs early in the course of HIV infection
- Syndrome 2: Gradual onset of abnormal sensation in the toes, feet, distal legs, and fingers: numbness, tingling, pins, and needles plus neuropathic pain is typical of this neuropathy, which occurs later in the course of the infection when AIDS has developed
- Syndrome 3: Abrupt to subacute onset of lower extremity motor and sensory dysfunction as well as bowel/bladder dysfunction is typical of the CMV-related polyradiculitis, which occurs late in the course, when AIDS has developed

Natural History

- Syndrome 1: Course typical for Guillain-Barré syndrome, including the response to customary therapies
- Syndrome 2: Slowly worsening deficits over years manifested by more proximal spread of the abnormal sensations
- Syndrome 3: Persisting, severe deficits, which only partially respond to antiviral treatment

Diagnosis

Differential diagnosis

- Other acute to chronic peripheral neuropathies
- Polyneuropathy related to the medications used to treat the HIV infection
- Myelopathies due to transverse myelitis, multiple sclerosis, spondylosis, epidural abscess, or late HIV infection

History

- Syndrome 1: Acute neuropathy developing over days to about 4 weeks, with motor and sensory deficits typical of Guillain-Barré syndrome
- Syndrome 2: Chronically evolving length-dependent sensory, and to a much lesser degree motor dysfunction, which occurs late in the course of HIV infection or in its treatment with antiretroviral medications
- Syndrome 3: Acute to subacute evolution of lower extremity weakness and sensory loss in the legs, accompanied by loss of urinary and rectal sphincter control

Physical examination

Syndromes 1 and 2

- Decreased sensation to vibratory, light touch, pin prick, or monofilament-type stimuli in toes and distal aspect of the feet
- Absence of ankle muscle stretch reflexes
- Weakness of toe abduction, flexion, or extension motions

- Weakness of ankle extension and flexion plus weakness of intrinsic hand muscles in more severe cases

Syndrome 3

- Exam findings are those of a cauda equina syndrome
- Loss of sensation in the feet, legs, and perineal area
- Weakness in foot and leg muscles, plus weakness of sphincters
- Loss of reflexes in the legs

Testing

- HIV antibody, HIV ribonucleic acid (RNA) titer (viral load), and CD4 count
- Hepatitis B antigen and antibody and hepatitis C antibody
- Fasting glucose and vitamin B12 levels
- Cerebrospinal fluid (CSF) analysis: Syndromes 1 and 3 show protein elevation typical of Guillain-Barré syndrome but also show an elevated white cell count
- CSF viral cultures may be positive for CMV in syndrome 3
- Syndrome 1: Nerve conduction studies show a "demyelinating pattern" with conduction velocity slowing below 70% of the low limit of normal and distal latency prolongation beyond 125% of the upper limit of normal. Lower and upper extremity nerves are involved
- Syndrome 2: Nerve conduction studies show an "axonal pattern" consisting of reduction of sensory response amplitudes in distal leg/foot nerves initially and then reduction of motor response amplitudes later. Conduction velocities become slowed but remain above 70% of the low limit of normal and distal latencies tend to not be abnormally prolonged. Upper extremities show lesser degrees of abnormality

- Syndrome 3: Lower extremity conduction studies show the pattern of a preganglionic lesion with motor studies showing low amplitude responses and only mildly slowed velocities. Sensory responses may remain normal. Needle EMG shows denervation in lower extremity muscles as well as the lumbar and possibly the lower thoracic paraspinal muscles. CSF analysis shows elevated white blood cells; protein and glucose may be low

Treatment

- Syndrome 1: Same as Guillain-Barré syndrome not related to HIV infection
- Syndrome 2: Optimal antiretroviral treatment of the HIV infection and symptomatic treatment of the paresthesias and neuropathic pain; consider altering antiretroviral medications for 2 to 3 months to distinguish neuropathy from HIV versus medication-related etiology
- Syndrome 3: CMV antivirals and rehabilitative management of the resulting paraplegia

Prognosis

- Syndrome 1: Course typical of Guillain-Barré syndrome not related to HIV infection
- Syndrome 2: Persistent to slowly worsening sensory and motor deficits
- Syndrome 3: Persistent, often severe, deficits in lower extremity and sphincter dysfunction

Suggested Readings

Amato A, Russell J. *Neuromuscular Disorders* (pp. 295–298). New York: McGraw Hill; 2008.

Hoffmann C, Gallant J. In: Nabel E, ed. *ACP Medicine*. [Section 7, Ch XXXIII]. Hamilton, ON, Canada: Decker; 2013.

Porphyric Neuropathy

John C. Kincaid MD

Description
Acute and potentially recurring polyneuropathy due to the metabolic disorder porphyria

Etiology
Genetic abnormalities in the pathway for the hepatic synthesis of heme cause episodic overproduction of neurotoxic intermediate components of heme

Epidemiology
- A very rare disorder in North America but knowledge of the condition is important due to it being frequently considered in the differential diagnosis of acute neuropathy
- Dominant inheritance pattern with a gene prevalence of between 1 in 1,000 to 100,000 in the white population for the acute intermittent variety of porphyria and 1 in 3000 in South African population where the variegated variety is most often encountered

Pathogenesis
Genetic abnormality in three enzymes of the hepatic heme synthesis pathway cause the porphyria syndromes that can produce peripheral neuropathy

- Porphobilinogen deaminase in the acute intermittent form
- Coproporphyrinogen oxidase in hereditary coproporphyria
- Protoporphyrinogen oxidase in variegate prophyria

Risk Factors
Having the genetic mutation and encountering biological conditions, which trigger overproduction of the prophyrin intermediates

- Medications which induce the cytochrome P450 system
- Fluctuation in gonadal hormone levels
- Biological or psychological stress
- Nutritional deprivation, which alters glucose metabolism

Clinical Features
- Relapsing attacks which begin in late adolescence and early adulthood
- Acute onset of abdominal pain, which may simulate an acute abdomen
- Psychiatric disturbance manifesting as agitation; hallucinations which appear in the same time frame as the abdominal pain
- Encephalopathy manifesting as seizures and at times coma
- Peripheral neuropathy, which begins several days after the abdominal pain
- Sun sensitivity in hereditary coproporphyria and variegated types, which produce blistering in sun exposed areas

Natural History
- Ten percent of attacks can be fatal
- The neuropathy improves over weeks to months after the acute attack but permanent deficits may occur

Diagnosis

Differential diagnosis
- Guillain-Barré syndrome
- Drug-induced neuropathy: chemotherapy, nitrofurantoin exposure
- Acute spinal cord syndrome: transverse myelitis or midline disk herniation

History
- Abrupt onset of abdominal pain
- Psychiatric disturbances concurrent with or shortly following the onset of abdominal pain
- Abrupt onset of peripheral neuropathy with features of:
  - Initial proximal predominance of the motor deficits, which may worsen over the course of days;
  - Cranial nerve involvement; and
  - Autonomic dysfunction with sympathetic overactivity, urinary hesitancy, and constipation
- Sensitivity to sun exposure with resulting blistering in the hereditary coproporphyria and variegated types

Physical examination
- Weakness which may be asymmetric initially but which may progress to generalized involvement, including the respiratory muscles

- Loss of muscle stretch reflexes proportionate to the pattern of weakness rather than the early generalized loss of reflexes typical of Guillain-Barré syndrome
- Deficits in limb and truncal sensory function such as light touch, vibration, and pin prick sensation are present if the patient's sensorium allows reliable examination
- Blistering skin lesions in sun exposed areas

Testing

- Assay of urine for presence of abnormally high concentrations of heme synthesis products:
  - Aminolevulinic acid
  - Porphobilinogen
- Assay of urine and stool for the presence of abnormally high concentrations of heme synthesis products:
  - Coproporphyin
  - Protophorphyrin
- Observe urine for change to dark color during exposure to light
- Nerve conduction studies show an "axonal" pattern of abnormality: motor and sensory response amplitudes are low if present, conduction velocities are no slower than the mid-30 meters per second range and distal latencies remain normal
- Needle EMG shows reduced motor unit potential recruitment initially and then signs of muscle membrane instability several weeks after onset
- Cerebrospinal fluid values tend to be normal or show only mild protein elevation

- Spinal cord or brain magnetic resonance imaging (MRI) does not show significant anatomical abnormalities
- Assay immediate family members for the presence of the biochemical abnormality

Treatment

- Supportive care, including respiratory support
- Elimination of potentially provocative medications (see the second reference for a comprehensive list and also visit www.porphyriafoundation.com)
- Morphine can be used for the abdominal pain
- Haloperidol can be used to treat agitation
- Propofol can be used to treat seizures
- Intravenous glucose administration (300–500 g/24 hrs) without insulin to suppress overproduction of heme intermediates
- Intravenous infusion of hematin at a 2 to 5 mg/kg/day dosing for 3 to 14 days suppresses production of aminolevulinic acid

Prognosis

- Improvement over a 2- to 12-month time frame
- Deficits in distal strength and sensory may persist

Suggested Readings

Anderson K, Kappas A. The porphyrias. In: Nabel E, ed. *ACP Medicine.* (Section 9, Chapter VII). Hamilton, ON, Canada: Decker; 2013.

Windebank A, Bonkovsky H. Porphyric neuropathy. In: Dyck PJ, Thomas PK, eds. *Peripheral Neuropathy.* 4th ed. (pp. 1883–1892). Philadelphia, PA: Elsevier; 2005.

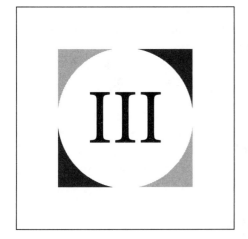

Neuromuscular Junction

Botulism

John C. Kincaid MD

Description

Syndrome of acutely evolving weakness of skeletal muscle and impairment of autonomic function due to peripheral cholinergic deficiency resulting from the effects of the toxin released by *Clostridium botulinum (C. botulinum)*

Etiology

- Exposure to the toxin produced by *C. botulinum*
- The most common source of the toxin is improperly sterilized homemade food products in which the bacteria grows and produces toxin
- Ingestion of *Clostridium* spores by infants and subsequent proliferation of the bacteria in the gastrointestinal tract may produce infantile botulism
- Wounds contaminated by soil can introduce the bacteria into the traumatized tissue and allow toxin in the wound site

Epidemiology

Rare but recognizable syndrome

- About 100 cases per year are reported in the United States
- Half of these come from western states where altitude and the resulting alteration of the boiling point of water may be a factor

Pathogenesis

- Botulinum toxin degrades several proteins in cholinergic nerve terminals, which play important roles in the docking of synaptic vesicles with the terminal membrane and release of neurotransmitters into the synaptic cleft
- The impaired release of acetylcholine produces deficits in somatic motor and autonomic functions

Risk Factors

- Exposure to food contaminated by *C. botulinum*
- Penetrating and crush injuries contaminated by soil
- Administration of illicit drugs by subcutaneous or intravenous route
- Ingestion of raw honey or other *Clostridium* spore-containing foods by infants

Clinical Features

- Onset of symptoms and signs 12 to 36 hours after exposure to the toxin
- Gastrointestinal (GI) disturbance in the form of nausea and vomiting and then constipation are the initial manifestations, with the exception of wound botulism in which GI disturbance does not occur
- Impairment of visual focusing and then development of diplopia
- Weakness of skeletal muscle, which may include muscles of respiration, that evolves over the next 2 to 4 days
- Absence of sensory disturbance

Natural History

- Deficits evolve to maximum over several days and then persist for several months

Diagnosis

Differential diagnosis

- Autoimmune myasthenia gravis
- Guillain-Barré syndrome
- Organophosphate poisoning
- Periodic paralysis
- Tick paralysis

History

- Onset of gastrointestinal disturbance, followed hours to a few days later by somatic muscle weakness, beginning several days after toxin exposure
- Maximal autonomic and skeletal muscle deficits result by 2 to 4 days after onset

Physical examination

- Look for a tick attached to the skin
- The sensorium should be normal in teenagers and adults; infants may appear lethargic due to the weakness
- Impaired pupillary reaction to light and accommodation
- Diplopia and weakness of other cranial muscles, followed hours to a few days later by weakness of the somatic muscles, including those of respiration

- The weakness may manifest with poor feeding and floppiness
- Muscle stretch reflexes are reduced or absent
- Sensory examination is normal

Testing

- Antiacetylcholine choline receptor antibodies will be negative
- The toxin may be present in serum, stool, or food samples
- Serum potassium, calcium, and magnesium levels should be normal
- Motor nerve and sensory conduction studies show normal conduction velocities and distal latencies but the motor response amplitude may be reduced
- Repetitive motor nerve stimulation may produce a decremental response at slow rates of stimulation but faster rates such as 10 to 20 Hz may be required
- An incremental response may be shown by repetitive stimulation at 30 to 50 Hz but if present, the amount of increment tends to be less than seen in Lambert-Eaton myasthenic syndrome; up to a 50% increment can be found in normal subjects due to pseudofacilitation
- Needle EMG may show abnormal resting activity in severely weak muscles several weeks after onset and may show somewhat small size motor unit potentials, which are unstable in configuration for one discharge to the next
- Cerebrospinal fluid protein levels tend to be normal

Treatment

- Supportive care, including intubation and ventilation
- The support may need to be maintained for weeks, as recovery requires the regeneration of motor and autonomic nerve terminals and synapses
- Trivalent antiserum to toxins A, B, and E should be administered when the diagnosis is strongly considered
- The antitoxin can be obtained from the Centers for Disease Control in Atlanta, GA, USA
- Verification of the absence of an allergy to the antitoxin should be verified by intradermal testing with horse serum, while monitoring for an allergic reaction
- Acetylcholinesterase inhibitors such as pyridostigmine may improve the weakness
- Occupational and physical therapy evaluation for optimization of functional capacity

Prognosis

- Improvement and eventual recovery should occur in the majority of patients who receive adequate management, including intensive care unit level care
- The duration of the need for highly supportive care may be weeks to a few months

Suggested Readings

Cherington M. Clinical spectrum of botulism. *Muscle Nerve.* 1998;21:701–710.

Chow A. Anaerobic Infections. In: Nabel E, ed. *ACP Medicine* (Section 7, Chapter V). Hamilton, ON, Canada: Decker; 2013.

Congenital Myasthenia Gravis

John C. Kincaid MD

Description

Syndromes due to genetic-based abnormalities in neuro-muscular junction structure and function, which present in newborns, infants, or children as episodes of fatigable weakness involving facial, limb, and respiratory muscles

Etiology

The congenital myasthenia gravis syndromes are classified by the site of functional abnormality:

- Presynaptic
- Synaptic
- Postsynaptic

Epidemiology

Very rare but recognizable syndromes: about 200 patients with these syndromes had been reported in literature by the mid-2000 time frame

Pathogenesis

Presynaptic abnormality:

- Choline acetyltransferase deficiency impairs the packaging of acetylcholine into synaptic vesicles and the replenishment of the vesicles during sustained muscle contraction
- This condition is also known as congenital myasthenic syndrome with episodic apnea

Synaptic abnormality:

- Congenital end plate acetylcholinesterase deficiency impairs breakdown of acetylcholine after release and results in persistent or recurrent opening of the acetylcholine receptor ion channel and impairment of repolarization of the postsynaptic membrane
- The deficiency of acetylcholinesterase arises due to an abnormality in collagen, which anchors the enzyme in the proper location of the postsynaptic membrane

Postsynaptic abnormality:

- These are the more common causes of congenital myasthenic syndrome
- Slow channel syndrome is due to alteration of the amino acid sequence of the ion channel proteins in the acetylcholine receptor and results in prolonged opening of the channel during synaptic transmission

- Fast channel syndrome is due to alteration of the normal amino acid sequence of the ion channel proteins in the acetylcholine receptor and results in shorter than normal opening of the channel during synaptic transmission

Risk Factors

Dominant inheritance in the slow channel syndrome, recessive inheritance in the others.

Clinical Features

- Onset in newborn or infant years is the more common clinical pattern
- Fatigable weakness of facial, limb, and at times respiratory muscles
- Static weakness may also develop in some syndromes

Natural History

- Defined by the specific syndrome: some produce episodic weakness, which lessens in severity as the patient enters teen to early adult years, whereas others produce a static to slowly progressive persistent weakness

Diagnosis

Differential diagnosis

- Autoimmune myasthenia gravis
- Infantile or juvenile motor neuron disease
- Muscular dystrophy with distal myopathy manifestations
- Botulism (for the initial episode of weakness)
- Periodic paralysis

History

- Recurring episodes of facial, limb, and at times, respiratory weakness
- Some attacks are precipitated by intercurrent illness such as infection
- A family history of similar attacks may be present

Physical examination

- Weakness of cranial and limb muscles which worsens with sustained use
- Persistent weakness of cranial, limb, and axial muscles in congenital acetylcholinesterase deficiency

- Episodic plus an underlying persistent weakness of neck extensors and the extensors of the wrist and fingers in slow channel syndrome

Testing

- Antiacetylcholine receptor and anti-muscle-specific tyrosine kinase antibodies will be negative
- Motor nerve and sensory conduction studies show normal conduction velocities and distal latencies
- Needle EMG should show normal resting activity and normal to small size motor unit potentials, which are unstable in configuration
- Repetitive motor nerve stimulation often shows a decremental response to 2 to 3 Hz stimuli, but this may not be present in each condition
- Patients with congenital acetylcholinesterase deficiency and slow channel syndrome demonstrate a repetitive (re-firing) component of the compound muscle action potential occurring 5 to 10 milliseconds after the negative phase of the potential following a single maximal stimulus
- Definitive diagnosis of the specific condition may require referral to a center with experience in the detailed analysis of these types of syndromes

Treatment

- Management of recurring episodes of acute respiratory failure may be required in congenital acetylcholinesterase deficiency

- Acetylcholinesterase inhibitors such as pyridostigmine may improve weakness in choline acetyltransferase deficiency and fast channel syndrome
- 3,4-Diaminopyridine may improve weakness in fast channel syndrome due to its enhancing effects on acetylcholine release from the nerve terminal
- Quinidine and fluoxetine may improve strength in slow channel syndrome
- Occupational and physical therapy evaluation for optimization of functional capacity

Prognosis

- Improvement in the frequency and severity of the episodes of weakness often occur as the infant moves into teen or early adult years
- Slowly worsening persistent weakness in neck extensors and wrist/finger extensor muscles occurs in slow channel syndrome

Suggested Readings

Engle A, Ohno K, Sine S. Congenital myasthenic syndromes in myology. In: Engle A, Franzini-Armstrong C, eds. 3rd ed. (pp. 1801–1844). New York: McGraw Hill; 2004.

Engle A, Shen X, Selcen D, Sine S. New horizons for congenital myasthenic syndromes. *Ann NY Acad Sci.* 2012;1275:54–62.

III: Neuromuscular Junction

Lambert-Eaton Myasthenic Syndrome

Cynthia L. Bodkin MD

Description

Lambert-Eaton Myasthenic Syndrome (LEMS) is an autoimmune disorder involving antibodies against the presynaptic neuromuscular junction

Etiology/Types

- Idiopathic
- About two thirds of cases are paraneoplastic disorder, of which roughly 90% are associated with small cell lung cancer

Epidemiology

- Rare disorder
- Mean age of onset is 54 years, with more than 80% older than 40 years
- Women are more prone to the idiopathic form, whereas men are more common in the paraneoplastic form

Pathogenesis

- Antibodies against P/Q voltage-gated calcium channels on the presynaptic terminal in 85% to 90% of patients
- About 74% of patients with lung cancer and 40% without cancer have antibodies to N-type calcium channels
- Acetylcholine release from the presynaptic terminal is impaired, leading to decreased activation of postsynaptic acetylcholine receptors on the muscle
- With fewer receptors activated, the endplate potentials may fall below threshold to generate an action potential

Risk Factors

- Autoimmune disease (rheumatoid arthritis, lupus, and inflammatory bowel disease)
- Small cell lung cancer
- Smoking

Clinical Features

- Fluctuating or fatigable weakness
- Temporary increased strength with short bursts of exercise
- Functional impairment out of proportion to objective weakness
- Proximal leg more than arm weakness
- Symptoms exacerbated by heat
- Stiffness and/or muscle aching is noted in one third of patients after physical activity
- Ocular and bulbar symptoms are not common
- Autonomic dysfunction, such as constipation, blurred vision, decreased sweating, and impotence, is common
- Respiratory failure from LEMS is rare

Natural History

- Symptoms often precede diagnosis of cancer by approximately 10 months (range 6 months to 4 years)

Diagnosis

Differential diagnosis

- Myasthenia syndrome
- Botulism
- Dermatomyositis/polymyositis
- Amyotrophic lateral sclerosis
- Electrolyte abnormality

History

- Fluctuating weakness
- Difficulty walking
- Dry mouth, eyes, or skin
- Constipation and/or urinary retention

Examination

- Variable muscle weakness with proximal muscles more involved than distal
- Decreased or absent deep tendon reflexes with initial testing, which improves with repetitive testing
- Mild ptosis or diplopia may be present in some patients
- Examination may be normal

Testing

- P/Q voltage-gated calcium channels antibodies
- N-type calcium channel antibodies
- Nerve conduction studies demonstrate decreased-to-normal absolute values of amplitude. Greater than 10% decrement can be seen at 2 to 3 Hz repetitive stimulation, whereas facilitation is noted with 20 to 50 Hz stimulation or short bursts of exercise
- Needle EMG demonstrates normal motor unit duration and amplitude but varying potentials in weak muscles

- Single-fiber electromyography demonstrates increase jitter and neuromuscular blocking
- Chest computed tomography (CT) scan, and positron emission tomography (PET) scan should be considered to evaluate for underlying cancer
- Bronchoscope for patients at risk for lung cancer

Pitfalls
- Delayed diagnosis
- Not screening for underlying cancer

Red flags
- Fasciculation and atrophy

Treatment

Medical
- Treat underlying cancer
- 3,4-diaminopyridine
- Anticholinesterase
- Immunosuppressive agents:
  - Corticosteroids
  - Azathioprine
  - Cyclosporine
- Plasmapheresis
- Intravenous immunglobulin

Surgical
- Surgical removal or biopsy of underlying cancer, if found

Consults
- Neurology
- Pulmonary
- Oncologist
- Physical medicine and rehabilitation

Complications of treatment
- Opportunistic infections
- Osteoporosis, weight gain, hyperglycemia, cataracts, and peptic ulcer in patients on steroids

Prognosis
- Dependent on underlying cancer and other autoimmune conditions

Helpful Hint
- Repeated screen for underlying cancer should be considered at interval periods

Suggested Readings

Amato AA, Russell JA. *Neuromuscular Disorders* (viii, pp. 457–528). New York: McGraw-Hill Medical; 2008.
Biller J. *Practical Neurology*. 4th ed. (pp. 559–569). Philadelphia, PA: Lippincott Williams & Wilkins, a Wolters Kluwer business; 2012.

III: Neuromuscular Junction

Myasthenia Gravis

Cynthia L. Bodkin MD

Description

Myasthenia gravis (MG) is an autoimmune disorder involving antibodies against the neuromuscular junction

Etiology/Types

- Idiopathic
- About 80% to 90% of patients have antibodies to acetylcholine (ACh) receptors (either modulating or blocking)
- About 25% of patients who do not have an antibody to (ACh) receptors will have antibodies to muscle-specific kinase (MuSK)
- Remainder is seronegative

Epidemiology

- Prevalence is approximately 1 in 10,000 to 20,000
- Male-to-female ratio estimated 1:2
- Age of onset can be any age with a peak in the 2nd and 3rd decade in women and 5th and 6th decade in men

Pathogenesis

- Antibodies to postsynaptic ACh receptors on the muscle decrease the number of receptors available to bind to ACh during nerve impulse. With fewer receptors available, the endplate potentials may fall below threshold to generate an action potential

Risk Factors

- Autoimmune disease (rheumatoid arthritis, lupus, and pernicious anemia in about 5%)
- Thyroid disease in about 10%
- Thymoma
- D-penicillamine and alfa-interferon therapy have induced MG

Clinical Features

- Fluctuating or fatigable weakness
- Half of patients will have ocular symptoms, either diplopia or ptosis
- Roughly 10% will present with leg weakness, 10% with generalized weakness, 10% with bulbar (dysarthria or dysphagia) weakness, and less than 1% with respiratory failure
- Symptoms tend to worsen later in the day and improve with physical rest
- Lack of autonomic dysfunction
- Urinary and bowl function usually remain normal

Natural History

- About 80% will develop ocular symptoms
- 80% to 85% of patients with ocular myasthenia will develop generalized weakness, most within the 1st year
- In 70% of patients the maximum weakness usually occurs within the first three years
- 10% to 15% can have a spontaneous remission

Diagnosis

Differential diagnosis

- Lambert-Eaton myasthenic syndrome
- Botulism
- Congenital myasthenic syndromes
- Compressive cranial neuropathies
- Mitochondrial cytopathies
- Oculopharyngeal muscular dystrophy
- Bulbar onset amyotrophic lateral sclerosis (ALS)
- Dermatomyositis/polymyositis

History

- The presentation can vary among patients but includes the following:
  - Fluctuating weakness
  - Diplopia and/or ptosis
  - Dysphagia and/or dysarthria
  - Weakness in legs/trouble walking
  - Shortness of breath or respiratory failure

Examination

- Variable muscle weakness with proximal muscles more involved than distal and arms more than legs
- Fluctuating asymmetrical extraocular movements
- Ptosis
- Nasal speech
- Neck extension weakness
- Exam may be normal

Testing

- ACh receptor antibodies
- Striated muscle antibody present in patients with thymoma
- MuSK antibody

- Nerve conduction studies demonstrate normal absolute values, but greater than 10% decrement can be seen at 2 to 3 Hz repetitive stimulation
- Needle EMG demonstrates normal motor unit duration and amplitude but varying potentials in weak muscles
- Single-fiber EMG demonstrates increased jitter and neuromuscular blocking
- Anticholinesterase tests with intravenous edrophonium can temporarily improve weakness. Patient must have an objective measurable abnormality on examination in order to measure improvement. Positive test can be seen in other neuromuscular disorders
- Antinuclear antibody
- Rheumatoid factor
- Thyroid stimulating hormone
- Chest computed tomography (CT) scan to evaluate for thymoma or thymic enlargement
- Magnetic resonance imaging (MRI) of brain and orbits for ocular myasthenia to evaluate for other potential causes

Pitfalls
- Delayed diagnosis
- Failure to recognize impending respiratory failure
- Temporary worsening with start of steroids can lead to respiratory failure

Red flags
- Pain
- Autonomic symptoms
- Fasciculation and atrophy

Treatment
Medical
- Anticholinesterase
- Immunosuppressive agents:
  - Corticosteroids
  - Azathioprine
  - Cyclosporine

- Plasmapheresis (common treatment with acute exacerbation)
- Intravenous immunoglobulin (common treatment with acute exacerbation)
- Supportive:
  - Close monitoring in intensive care unit for patients in a crisis
  - Bi-level positive airway pressure
  - Intubation
  - Feeding tube

Surgical
- Thymectomy for patients with a thymoma and can be considered in patients without a thymoma

Consults
- Neurology
- Pulmonary
- Speech pathology
- Dietitian

Complications of treatment
- Opportunistic infections
- Risk of lymphoproliferative malignancies
- Osteoporosis, weight gain, hyperglycemia, cataracts, and peptic ulcer in patients on steroids

Prognosis
- Variable:
  - Mortality from MG is unusual due to the current advancements in medical care
- In 70% of patients the maximum weakness usually occurs within the first 3 years
- 10% to 15% can have a spontaneous remission

Helpful Hint
- Steroids may temporarily worsen weakness

Suggested Readings
Amato AA, Russell JA. *Neuromuscular Disorders* (viii, pp. 457–528). New York: McGraw-Hill Medical; 2008.
Biller J. *Practical Neurology*. 4th ed. (pp. 559–569). Philadelphia, PA: Lippincott Williams & Wilkins, a Wolters Kluwer business; 2012.

III: Neuromuscular Junction

Organophosphate Poisoning

John C. Kincaid MD

Description

Syndrome of acute overactivity of cholinergic synaptic transmission due to blockade of acetylcholinesterase by organophosphate compounds, with resulting central nervous system, autonomic nervous system, and neuromuscular manifestations

Etiology

Exposure to the causative compounds by contact with excessive amounts of insecticides, contaminants of food products, or exposure to nerve agent warfare compounds in military or terrorist settings

Epidemiology

The most common source of this type of exposure is suicide attempts in which ingestion of insecticides occurs.

Pathogenesis

- Carbamate and organophosphate compounds inhibit the activity of acetyl cholinesterase, resulting in excess acetylcholine at synapses in the central and autonomic nervous system and at the neuromuscular junction
- Manifestations of the excess cholinergic activity include encephalopathy, seizures, miosis, excessive salivation, bronchospasm, abdominal cramping, hyperhidrosis, fasciculations, and muscular weakness
- Delayed manifestations of myelopathy or peripheral neuropathy due to the compounds' effects on structural proteins of central and peripheral nerves may occur in survivors of the acute exposure

Risk Factors

Exposure to organophosphate compounds in the form of high dose contact with insecticides such as malathion, ingestion of food products contaminated by industrial lubricating agents such as triorthocresyl phosphates, or contact with nerve gas warfare agents such as soman, sarin, or VX in weapon storage, terrorist, or military action-type settings

Clinical Features

- Acute onset of abdominal cramps, vomiting, diarrhea, hyperhidrosis, and excessive salivation
- Depending on the compound, additional manifestations may include muscular weakness up to the degree of respiratory paralysis and central nervous system manifestations of agitation, encephalopathy, and seizures
- Survivors of the acute exposure may develop peripheral neuropathy and myelopathy weeks later

Natural History

- Prompt treatment in a hospital or military triage setting permits survival
- Longer-term effects such as peripheral neuropathy or myelopathy may not be preventable

Diagnosis

Differential diagnosis

- Status epilepticus of other etiology
- Acute abdomen
- Opioid withdrawal
- Myasthenic crisis
- Attack of porphyria
- Encephalitis

History

- Acute onset of gastrointestinal disturbance shortly after exposure to or ingestion of the compound
- Seizures and muscular paralysis follow minutes later

Physical examination

- Signs of cholinergic excess: hyperhydrosis, miosis, sialorrhea, fasciculations
- Altered sensorium
- Generalized convulsions
- Weakness of skeletal muscles

Testing

- Chest radiograph, blood gas, electrocardiogram, electrolytes, calcium, and magnesium levels
- Computed tomography (CT) of the head
- Electroencephalogram

Treatment

- Clothing removal and decontamination of skin
- Protection of rescue and medical workers with respirators, butyl rubber gloves rather than latex, butyl rubber aprons
- Supportive care, including intubation and ventilation
- Gastric lavage if ingestion has occurred

- Administration of atropine and 2-PAM (1–2 g IV immediately followed by 200–500 mg/hr) to counteract cholinergic excess
- Military personnel in war settings carry atropine and 2-PAM injectors
- Seek input from a poison control center

Prognosis

- Survival is possible if recognition of the scenario is prompt and treatment is instituted

- Peripheral neuropathy and myelopathy may develop weeks after the acute event in survivors

Suggested Readings

Holstege C, Kirk M, Sidell F. Chemical warfare nerve agent poisoning. *Crit Care Clin.* 1997;13:923–942.

Wiegland T, Patel M, Olson K. Management of poisoning and drug overdose. In: Nabel E, ed. *ACP Medicine.* (Section 8, Chapter I). Hamilton, ON, Canada: Decker; 2013.

III: Neuromuscular Junction

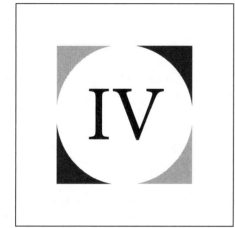

Radiculopathies/ Plexopathies

Brachial Plexopathy

Gentry Dodd MD ■ Nathan D. Prahlow MD

Description

A pathologic process affecting a group of nerves in the brachial plexus, usually distal to the dorsal root ganglion and proximal to the peripheral nerves

Etiology

- Trauma:
  - Stretching of nerves
  - Nerve transection
  - Obstetric injuries
  - Hemorrhage
- Cancer:
  - Direct tumor invasion
  - Radiation therapy
- Idiopathic:
  - Neuralgic amyotrophy

Types

- Upper plexus lesions
  - For example, Erb's palsy
- Lower trunk lesions
  - For example, Klumpke's palsy

Epidemiology

- 0.4% of patients with cancer
- 2% to 5% of cancer patients treated with radiation
- Traumatic brachial plexus injuries usually occur in young males (89%)
  - Age range is 14 to 63 years, with a mean of 29 years
- Idiopathic brachial plexopathy (Neuralgic Amyotrophy) has an annual incidence of 2 to 3 per 100,000
- Iatrogenic causes are usually from positioning in surgery or anesthesia

Pathogenesis

- Nerve compression or traction from trauma, such as would be experienced with a direct blow to the shoulder during contact sports, can lead to nerve damage or even transection
- Inflammatory, metabolic, and radiation-induced plexopathies often involve small vessel ischemia
- Metabolic abnormalities, such as diabetes, can cause local inflammation and focal ischemia
- Neoplasms can place direct pressure on the plexus but more often causes a plexopathy via direct nerve or connective tissue invasion

Risk Factors

- Trauma to the shoulder, causing a downward force, with possible movement of the head and neck to the contralateral side, can cause traction to the upper brachial plexus
- Traction to the arm, such as attempting to catch one's self while falling, can lead to lower plexus injury
- Diabetes (although lumbosacral plexopathies are more common)
- Tumors of the head, neck, and chest
- History of radiation therapy to the upper chest, neck, or shoulder

Clinical Features

- Pain, either acute or progressive, in the shoulder or upper arm
- Evolving arm, shoulder, or hand numbness
- Weakness of the upper extremity
- Atrophy, likely to not be appreciated until several weeks after plexus injury
- Sympathetic changes can be seen with a C8, T1 lesion

Natural History

- Traumatic etiology:
  - Most natural improvements occur within 6 months
  - In general, recovery is poor
  - Injuries that have a degree of axonal continuity have a more favorable outcome
- Nerve pain may be severe and can persist for a long time

Diagnosis

Differential diagnosis

- Radiculopathy
- Rotator cuff disease
- Shoulder dislocation
- Thoracic outlet syndrome

History

- Trauma
- History of head/neck cancer with or without targeted radiation therapy
- Sensory disturbances
- Focal upper extremity weakness

Exam

- Manual muscle testing
- Sensory testing
- Deep tendon reflexes
- Evaluate for specific arm/hand positioning:
  - Erb's palsy—extended arm, pronated forearm, flexed hand:
    - "Waiter's tip" position
    - C5, C6 injury
  - Klumpke's palsy—claw hand:
    - C8, T1 injury
- Look for signs of atrophy in the upper extremities

Testing

- Computed tomography (CT) myelography
- Magnetic resonance imaging (MRI) without contrast
- Plain films to look for bony structural abnormalities
- EMG—should be performed 3 to 6 weeks after injury
  - Sensory nerve action potentials may be normal if the lesion is preganglionic (proximal to the dorsal root ganglion)
  - Sensory potentials will be abnormal if the lesion is postganglionic
  - EMG demonstrates normal paraspinal activity with peripheral abnormalities

Pitfalls

- Contracture deformities can develop and are difficult to treat

Red flags

- Once muscle atrophy is present, regaining full functional capacity is difficult

Treatment

Medical

- Medications to control pain:
  - Non-steroidal anti-inflammatory drugs (NSAIDs)
  - Anticonvulsants:
    - Gabapentin
    - Lyrica
  - Tricyclic antidepressants:
    - Nortriptyline
    - Amitriptyline
  - Cymbalta is often used as an adjunctive therapy to help treat neuropathic pain
    - Opioids in general are not useful for the treatment of neuropathic pain
- If the cause of plexopathy is due to diabetes or renal disease, the underlying comorbidities should also be treated appropriately

Exercise

- Range-of-motion exercises to prevent contractures and secondary deformities, followed by gravity assisted exercise, then resistance exercise
- Passive muscle stretching helps prevent muscle atrophy
- Electrical stimulation to the denervated muscles can help prevent significant atrophy

Modalities

- Electrical stimulation (E-stim) for pain control
- Transcutaneous electrical nerve stimulation; although efficacy is questionable in chronic and neuropathic pain
- Ultrasound for deep pain and muscle spasm

Injections

- Focal nerve block

Surgical treatment

- Nerve/plexus reconstruction
- Spinal cord stimulator placement
- Deep brain stimulator
- Lesioning of the dorsal root entry zone

Consults

- Physiatry
- Neurology
- Neurosurgery

Complications of treatment

- Surgery may not completely reverse symptomatology
- Placement of spinal cord stimulators and deep brain stimulators are associated with the usual risks as well as intracranial/intradural infections

Prognosis

- A good recovery can be expected if the cause is identified and treated appropriately
  - For example, head/neck cancer
- Limited muscle movement may be seen months after the damage
- Surgical intervention may not show significant results until 3 to 4 years after initial treatment and following significant intensive therapy

Helpful Hint

- If an EMG demonstrates normal sensory action potentials, there may still be a nerve root avulsion

Suggested Readings

Simmons Z. Electrodiagnosis of brachial plexopathies and proximal upper extremity neuropathies. *Phys Med Rehab Clin N Am.* 2013; 24(1):13–32.

Wilbourn AJ. Plexopathies. *Neurol Clin.* 2007;25(1):139–171.

IV: Radiculopathies/Plexopathies

Lumbosacral Plexopathy

Gentry Dodd MD ■ Nathan D. Prahlow MD

Description
A pathologic process affecting a group of nerves in the lumbosacral plexus, usually distal to the dorsal root ganglion and proximal to the peripheral nerves

Etiology
- Trauma:
  - Stretching of nerves
  - Nerve transection
  - Hemorrhage/hematoma
- Cancer:
  - Direct tumor invasion
  - Radiation therapy

Types
- Lumbar plexus lesions:
  - Involves the anterior rami of L2–L4
- Sacral plexus lesions:
  - Involves the anterior rami of L5–S3

Epidemiology
- For diabetics, the incidence of a proximal neuropathy is 8 per 1000
- In traumatic cases with a sacral fracture, there is a 2% incidence of lumbosacral plexopathy
  - With other pelvic fractures, the incidence is 0.8%
- One per 2000 to 6000 obstetric deliveries result in lumbosacral plexopathies
- Idiopathic cases of lumbosacral plexopathy are rare, with only a few hundred cases in the literature

Pathogenesis
- Nerve compression or transection from trauma
- Inflammatory, metabolic, and radiation induced plexopathies often involve small vessel ischemia
- Metabolic abnormalities, such as diabetes, can cause local inflammation and focal ischemia
- Neoplasms can place direct pressure on the plexus but more often causes a plexopathy via direct nerve or connective tissue invasion
- Hip dislocations can cause direct trauma to the plexus
- Retroperitoneal hematomas can place pressure on the plexus

Risk Factors
- Trauma to the pelvis or hip, such as seen with motor vehicle accidents or gunshot wounds
- Diabetes—lumbosacral plexopathies are more common than brachial plexopathies as a result of diabetes
- Tumors of the pelvis or hip
- History of radiation therapy to the pelvis or thigh regions

Clinical Features
- Pain, either acute or progressive, in the pelvis, thigh, or lower extremity
- Evolving thigh, leg, calf, or foot numbness
- Weakness of the lower extremity
- Atrophy, likely to not be appreciated until several weeks after plexus injury

Natural History
- Traumatic etiology:
  - Most natural improvements occur within 6 months
  - In general, recovery is poor
  - Injuries having a degree of axonal continuity have a more favorable outcome
- Nerve pain may be severe and persist for a long time

Diagnosis

Differential diagnosis
- Radiculopathy
- Polyradiculopathy (cauda equina syndrome)
- Anterior horn cell disease:
  - Painless, diffuse weakness
  - Muscular atrophy
- Myopathy

History
- Trauma
- History of lower abdominal/pelvic cancer with or without targeted radiation therapy
- Sensory disturbances
- Focal lower extremity weakness

Examination
- Manual muscle testing
- Sensory testing
- Deep tendon reflexes
- Specific examination findings depend on which portion of the plexus is involved
  - Lumbar involvement:
    - Weakness of hip flexion, knee extension, thigh adduction

- Decreased sensation of the anteromedial thigh
- Decreased patellar reflex
  - Sacral involvement:
    - Weakness of hip extension, hip abduction, knee flexion, ankle plantar flexion and dorsiflexion
    - Decreased sensation in the posterior thigh and plantar surface of the foot
    - Decreased Achilles reflex
- Look for signs of atrophy in the lower extremities

Testing
- Computed tomography (CT) myelography
- Magnetic resonance imaging (MRI) without contrast
- Plain films to look for bony structural abnormalities
- EMG—should be performed 3 to 6 weeks postinjury
  - Sensory and motor nerve action potential amplitudes are reduced, indicating a lesion distal to the dorsal root ganglion
    - Sensory potentials will be abnormal if the lesion is postganglionic
  - EMG can demonstrate denervation, as evidenced by fibrillations and positive sharp waves, as well as reduced recruitment
    - For the diagnosis, denervation needs to be observed in muscles that are innervated by two different lumbosacral spinal levels that involve at least two different peripheral nerves

Pitfalls
- Once muscle atrophy is present, regaining full functional capacity is difficult

Red flags
- Cancer-related history must be elicited

Treatment
Medical treatment
- Medications to control pain:
  - Non-steroidal anti-inflammatory drugs (NSAIDs)
  - Anticonvulsants:
    - Gabapentin
    - Lyrica
  - Tricyclic antidepressants:
    - Nortriptyline
    - Amitriptyline
  - Cymbalta is often used as an adjunctive therapy to help treat neuropathic pain
    - Opioids in general are not useful for the treatment of neuropathic pain

- If the cause of plexopathy is due to diabetes, any underlying comorbidities should also be treated appropriately

Exercise
- Range-of-motion exercises to prevent contractures and secondary deformities
  - Followed by gravity-assisted exercise then resistance exercise
- Passive muscle stretching helps prevent muscle atrophy
- Electrical stimulation to the denervated muscles can help prevent significant atrophy

Modalities
- Electrical stimulation (E-stim) for pain control
  - Transcutaneous electrical nerve stimulation; although efficacy is questionable in chronic and neuropathic pain
- Ultrasound for muscle spasm and pain control

Injections
- Focal nerve block

Surgical treatment
- Nerve/plexus reconstruction
- Spinal cord stimulator placement
- Deep brain stimulator
- Lesioning of the dorsal root entry zone

Consults
- Physiatry
- Neurology
- Neurosurgery

Complications of treatment
- Surgery may not completely reverse symptomatology
- Placement of spinal cord stimulators and deep brain stimulators are associated with the usual risks as well as intracranial/intradural infections

Prognosis
- A good recovery can be expected if the cause is identified and treated appropriately
- Limited muscle movement may be seen months after the damage

Helpful Hint
- If an EMG demonstrates normal sensory action potentials, there may be a nerve root avulsion

Suggested Reading
Wilbourn AJ. Plexopathies. *Neurol Clin.* 2007;25(1):139–171.

IV: Radiculopathies/Plexopathies

Neuralgic Amyotrophy (Parsonage-Turner Syndrome)

Gentry Dodd MD ■ Nathan D. Prahlow MD

Description

Neuralgic amyotrophy, also known as Parsonage-Turner Syndrome (PTS) and idiopathic brachial plexopathy, is a disorder consisting of a constellation of findings usually preceded by abrupt onset of upper extremity/shoulder pain followed by progressive motor weakness, dysesthesia, and numbness.

Etiology

■ Can be triggered by the following:
- Infection
- Surgery/anesthesia
- Rheumatic disease:
  • Connective tissue disorders
  • Systemic lupus erythematosis
  • Polyarteritis nodosa
- Trauma:
  • Remote from the shoulder girdle complex
- Immunizations:
  • Tetanus
  • Diphtheria, pertussis, tetanus (DPT)
  • Smallpox

Types

■ No specific types of PTS exist, but varying portions of the plexus may be affected

Epidemiology

■ Overall, the incidence of neuralgic amyotrophy is 1.64 per 100,000; however, this may be underreported, as this is a difficult clinical diagnosis
■ The incidence is higher in men than women, with ratios ranging from 11:9 to 11:1
■ There is no apparent left or right side preference; bilateral involvement occurs in up to 30% of patients
■ Affected age groups range from 3 months to 75 years, with the highest prevalence in the 3rd to 7th decades

Pathogenesis

■ The pathology of this idiopathic disorder is not clearly understood, but there are several theories as to the cause of the sudden onset of acute shoulder pain
- Viral illness may directly affect the brachial plexus

- An autoimmune response to a virus may directly affect the brachial plexus
- Vasculitic disease, such as polyarteritis nodosa, systemic lupus erythematosus, and temporal arteritis, which are related to neuralgic amyotrophy suggest that a vascular component is at play
- Inflammatory or mechanically induced ischemia may be the cause of the sudden onset of pain
  • Perineural thickening and neovascularization have been reported in nerve biopsies
■ Cases related to surgery are often thought to be due to either poor positioning that results in brachial plexus traction or immune-mediated inflammation of the brachial plexus

Risk Factors

■ The most commonly described risk factor is viral illness, with approximately 25% of patients with neuralgic amyotrophy having had a preceding viral illness
■ Recent immunization is the second most commonly cited risk factor: Up to 15% of patients with neuralgic amyotrophy had a recent immunization prior to the development of this syndrome

Clinical Features

■ Sudden onset of constant, severe shoulder pain that may extend to the trapezius, forearm, and hand
- Usually, no constitutional signs or symptoms are associated with shoulder pain, although a viral illness may precede the initial presentation
- The duration of pain usually lasts from days to weeks
- Pain is typically neuropathic in nature
■ Muscle weakness, atrophy, and sensory loss develop as the pain subsides and can last up to years
- Subtle muscular weakness can be seen days to weeks after initial symptom onset
- Obvious weakness and atrophy is usually seen within a month
- Scapular winging may be seen if the long thoracic nerve is involved

Natural History

- A study looking at functional strength revealed only 89% recovery within 3 years
- One-third of patients suffer from chronic pain and functional deficits up to 6 years after initial diagnosis

Diagnosis

Differential diagnosis

- Rotator cuff disease
- Cervical disc disease
- Bicipital tendonitis
- Other causes of brachial plexopathy

History

- Recent surgical intervention or anesthesia
- Viral illness preceding the onset of shoulder pain
- Immunization shortly before shoulder pain began

Examination

- Manual muscle testing
- Sensory testing
- Deep tendon reflexes
- Visual inspection looking for signs of muscle atrophy

Testing

- The diagnosis is largely a clinical one
- Chest x-ray to rule out potential mass or Pancoast tumor
- Cervical spine magnetic resonance imaging (MRI) is helpful in ruling out cervical disc disease as the potential etiologic agent
  - This, however, can cloud the clinical picture given the many incidental, nonclinically important findings that can be seen in advanced imaging
- EMG—should be performed 3 to 6 weeks after injury
  - Sensory and motor nerve action potential amplitudes of distal muscles are commonly normal as the proximal muscles are more often affected
  - EMG can demonstrate positive sharp wave and fibrillations, signs of acute denervation, 3 to 4 weeks after symptom onset
    - This is seen in peripheral nerves and nerve root distributions, as opposed to just nerve root distribution (as seen in radiculopathy)
  - EMG performed 3 to 4 months after symptom onset may show chronic denervation with signs of early reinnervation (polyphasia)
  - There may be contralateral EMG abnormalities even without symptoms

Pitfalls

- If EMG abnormalities are seen in a nerve root distribution only and not also in a peripheral nerve distribution, the likely etiology of shoulder pain is radiculopathy

Red flags

- Shooting arm pain is typically a sign of radiculopathy rather than neuralgic amyotrophy

Treatment

Medical

- The best treatment at this time remains unknown
- There is some evidence to suggest that oral corticosteroids administered during the acute pain phase of neuralgic amyotrophy can shorten the duration of intense pain and expedite motor recovery
- Because the acute pain phase of neuralgic amyotrophy is usually short in duration—days to weeks—non-steroidal anti-inflammatory drugs (NSAIDs) and opioids are generally recommended over the use of tricyclics and anticonvulsants given their delayed onset in pain relieving effect
- Immunotherapy has been used in the past as a potential therapeutic agent, although there are a limited number of studies available to demonstrate its effectiveness

Exercise

- Range-of-motion exercises to prevent contractures and secondary deformities
  - Followed by gravity-assisted exercise and then resistance exercise
  - Strength training should be delayed until significant reinnervation of the affected muscles has developed
- Electrical stimulation to the denervated muscles can help prevent significant atrophy

Modalities

- Electrical stimulation (E-stim) for pain control
- Transcutaneous electrical nerve stimulation for pain control

Injections

- No specific injection techniques exist for the treatment of neuralgic amyotrophy

Surgical Treatment

- No specific surgical interventions exist for the treatment of neuralgic amyotrophy, although chronic pain can be treated in several ways
  - Spinal cord stimulator
  - Dorsal root entry zone lesioning

IV: Radiculopathies/Plexopathies

Consults
- Physiatry
- Neurology

Complications of treatment
- If resistance exercises are begun before adequate reinnervation is begun, axonal regeneration and subsequent muscle reinnervation may be retarded
  - A follow-up EMG can help demonstrate the degree of reinnervation of the affected muscles

Prognosis
- Prognosis for functional recovery is usually good in most cases
- One study suggested an 89% functional recovery in patients 3 years after symptom onset
  - This study looked only at functional recovery and not EMG findings of reinnervation, so recovery may be exaggerated as there can be muscular compensation
- Reinnervation usually begins 6 months to 1 year after initial injury

Helpful Hint
- Diagnosis is made by the acute onset of severe pain, followed by resolution of pain, which is in turn followed by muscle weakness and atrophy

Suggested Reading
Tjoumakaris FP, Anakwenze OA, et al. Neuralgic amyotrophy (Parsonage-Turner syndrome). *J Am Acad Ortho Surg.* 2012;20(7):443–449.

Radiculopathy

Gentry Dodd MD ■ Nathan D. Prahlow MD

Description
Radiculopathies are pathologic processes that affect the spinal nerve at the root level that often present as pain radiating into an extremity

Etiology
- Spondylosis
- Disk herniation
- Diabetes
- Infection
- Tumor: lipoma, meningioma, neurofibroma
- Infarction
- Arachnoiditis: from surgery, anesthesia, myelogram

Types
- Cervical
- Thoracic
- Lumbar

Epidemiology
- Cervical:
  - Mean age at diagnosis is 47.9 years
  - Incidence rates of 63.5 and 107.3 per 100,000 for men and women, respectively
  - Male:female ratio of 1.7:1
  - C7 accounts for roughly 70% of all cervical radiculopathy cases, C6 20%, and the remaining 10% between C5, C8, and T1
- Thoracic:
  - Up to 5% of symptomatic herniated discs occur in the thoracic region
  - Equal rates between men and women
- Lumbar:
  - Equal rates between men and women
  - Majority of lesions involve the L5 and S1 roots

Pathogenesis
- Compressive:
  - Bony overgrowth and degenerative changes in the vertebral joints can lead to neuroforaminal narrowing and compression of the nerve roots
  - Disc herniation can also cause nerve root compression if the herniation occurs laterally

- Noncompressive:
  - Noncompressive causes can lead to nerve root infarction or invasion that usually affects the sensory portion of the nerve root
- Cervical radiculopathies are usually due to bony issues, whereas those of the lumbar spine are more often caused by disc herniation

Risk Factors
- Trauma
- History of degenerative disc or joint disease

Clinical Features
- Pain in the neck, arms, trunk, legs, or back
- Potentially atypical pain that presents as chest pain, breast pain, or facial pain for cervical radiculopathy
- Numbness or dysesthesia that occurs in a more-or-less typical nerve root distribution pattern
- Weakness

Natural History
- In general, the majority of radiculopathy cases are self-limited and respond well to conservative therapy without the need for interventional or surgical treatment.

Diagnosis

Differential diagnosis
- Peripheral entrapment neuropathy
- Brachial/lumbosacral plexopathy
- Spinal stenosis
- Cauda equina syndrome

History
- Abrupt onset of symptoms is seen more commonly with a herniated disc
- If the radiculopathy is caused by spondylosis, symptom onset is more gradual

Examination
- Sensory testing
- Upper and lower limb strength and reflex testing
- Observation for atrophy

IV: Radiculopathies/Plexopathies

109

- Spurling's maneuver—extend and rotate the neck toward the symptomatic side with a downward compression. This test is positive with a reproduction in radiating pain symptoms. Spurling's maneuver is very specific, but not all that sensitive
- Straight leg raise test with reproduction of radicular symptoms
- Bowstring sign is a relief of radicular pain with flexing of the knee during the straight leg raise test

Testing
- Noncontrast magnetic resonance imaging (MRI), most helpful when surgery is being considered
- Computed tomography (CT) myelography when MRI is contraindicated; certain cases may require in addition to MRI testing
- Plain films can help establish the extent of spondylosis
- EMG:
  - Nerve conduction studies and EMG must be performed together
  - Sensory nerve action potentials are normal
  - Motor action potentials may have decreased amplitudes
  - EMG should be performed in three muscles of the same myotome with different peripheral innervations
    - Motor units may have increased duration, amplitude, and polyphasia with decreased recruitment
    - Positive sharp waves and fibrillations appear in the periphery in about 3 to 6 weeks

Pitfalls
- Missing a conus medularis lesion or myelopathy
- Presence or absence of bowel and bladder complaints may be misleading

Red flags
- Progressive weakness
- Difficulty walking and bowel/bladder dysfunction are suggestive of myelopathy
- A history of fever, chills, unexplained weight loss, and intravenous drug abuse should cause concern that tumor or infection is active
- An increase in symptoms when lying down is suggestive of a dural mass

Treatment

Medical
- Avoidance of exacerbating activities
- Non-steroidal anti-inflammatory drugs (NSAIDs)

- Oral analgesics
- Short course of oral steroid medication

Exercise
- Physical therapy referrals should focus on range-of-motion and strengthening exercises

Modalities
- Traction to the cervical and lumbar spines can result in relief of nerve root compression
  - Traction is not recommended for cases involving spinal cord compression or large disc protrusion, especially central cervical herniated discs
- The efficacy of traction in the treatment of radiculopathy is unclear

Injections
- Epidural steroid infections are most effective when the etiology is a herniated disc
- Caudal epidural steroid injections are most beneficial for S1 nerve root lesions

Surgical treatment
- Should be reserved for cases that do not respond to an adequate trial of conservative treatment (usually 6–12 weeks) or if there is presence of progressive motor weakness
- Cervical:
  - Anterior cervical discectomy and fusion
  - Posterior laminoforaminotomy, used when a single lateral disc herniation is present
- Lumbar:
  - Laminectomy
  - Discectomy

Consults
- Physiatry
- Neurology
- Neurosurgery

Complications of treatment
- Medication side effects
- Potential for intravascular or intraspinal injections with interventional procedures
- Abnormalities seen on imaging do not always correlate with symptoms, and patients can be referred for unnecessary surgery
- Surgical complications: failed back surgery syndrome, chronic pain, and arachnoiditis

Prognosis

■ In the absence of worsening symptoms, increasing muscle weakness, bowel or bladder dysfunction, the majority of cases resolve with conservative measures in 2 to 3 months

Helpful Hint

■ Until the diagnosis is confirmed by EMG, fluoroscopically guided injection, or surgery, one should describe the symptoms of "radiating limb pain," rather than label the patient with the term "radiculopathy."

Suggested Readings

Chiodo A, Haig AJ. Lumbosacral radiculopathies: Conservative approaches to management. *Phys Med Rehabil Clin N Am.* 2002;13(3):609–621, viii.

Wilbourn AJ, Aminoff MJ. AAEM minimonograph 32: The electrodiagnostic examination in patients with radiculopathies. American Association of Electrodiagnostic Medicine. *Muscle Nerve.* 1998;21(12):1612–1631.

Wolff MW, Levine LA. Cervical radiculopathies: Conservative approaches to management. *Phys Med Rehabil Clin N Am.* 2002;13(3):589–608, vii.

IV: Radiculopathies/Plexopathies

Thoracic Outlet Syndrome—Neurogenic

Nathan D. Prahlow MD

Description
A disputed syndrome of upper limb symptoms, including radiating pain, paresthesias, and weakness, due to the compression of the neurovascular bundle superior to the first rib and posterior to the clavicle

Etiology/Types
- Neurogenic
- Arterial
- Venous

Epidemiology
- 10 cases per 100,000 people
- >90% neurogenic
- <1% arterial

Pathogenesis
- Brachial plexus compression from the scalene muscles

Risk Factors
- Cervical rib found in <1% of the population (70% seen in women); most are asymptomatic
- Cervical rib predisposes to symptom development after neck trauma

Clinical Features
- Neck and arm pain
- Arm paresthesias
- Upper limb weakness
- Occipital headaches

Natural History
- May develop after neck trauma, such as whiplash-type injuries

Diagnosis
Differential diagnosis
- Cervical radiculopathy
- Brachial plexopathy
- Arterial thoracic outlet syndrome (TOS)
- Venous TOS
- Posterior shoulder girdle myofascial pain syndrome
- Ulnar neuropathy

History
- Neck trauma
- Limb pain
- Paresthesias
- Shoulder/arm/hand weakness
- Neck pain
- Occipital headaches
- May have symptoms of Raynaud's phenomenon

Examination
- Neck rotation with side-bending to elicit pain/paresthesias in contralateral limb
- Tenderness on palpation of scalene muscles
- Symptoms brought on within 60 seconds of placing arm in 90 degrees abduction and full external rotation
- Modified Upper Limb Tension Test of Elvey: Abduct both shoulders to 90 degrees with extended elbows (causes ipsilateral symptoms), then dorsiflex both wrists (may increase ipsilateral symptoms), then tilt head to side—ear to shoulder (causes contralateral symptoms)
- Check pulses—normal in neurogenic, may be absent in arterial

Testing
- Cervical plain films: rule out cervical rib
- EMG: typically normal, but may have nonspecific abnormalities. Medial antebrachial cutaneous sensory, median motor, ulnar motor, and ulnar sensory studies may be abnormal

Pitfalls
- Adson's Test is of little to no clinical value in any type of TOS

Red flags
- Raynaud's phenomenon may cause confusion with arterial TOS

Treatment
Medical treatment
- Little evidence to support a specific treatment
- Consider the options listed below, based on the physician and patient preference

Exercise

- Restore cervical spine range of motion and shoulder/arm function
- Correct posture

Modalities

- Cervical traction
- Heat for muscle spasm/pain

Injection

- Botulinum toxin injection into scalene muscles

Surgical

- First cervical rib resection
- Supraclavicular neuroplasty of the brachial plexus

Consults

- Electromyography
- Thoracic surgery
- Neurosurgery

Complications of treatment

- Complications of therapies, modalities, and any medications utilized

- Surgery: incisional pain, pneumothorax, intercostalbrachial neuralgia, wound infection, wound hematoma

Prognosis

- Unknown
- Rare surgery
- May require several opinions and consults from TOS experts

Helpful Hint

- Specifically include the study of the medial antibrachial cutaneous sensory nerve if referring for EMG/NCS

Suggested Readings

Povlsen B, Belzberg A, Hansson T, et al. Treatment for thoracic outlet syndrome (Review). The Cochrane Collaboration. Indianapolis, IN: J Wiley & Sons; 2010.

Sanders RJ, Hammond SL, Rao NM. Diagnosis of thoracic outlet syndrome. *J Vascular Surg.* 2007;46(3): 601–604.

IV: Radiculopathies/Plexopathies

Thoracic Outlet Syndrome—Vascular

Nathan D. Prahlow MD

Description
A disputed syndrome of upper limb symptoms, including radiating pain, paresthesias, and weakness, due to the compression of the neurovascular bundle superior to the first rib and posterior to the clavicle

Etiology/Types
- Neurogenic
- Arterial
- Venous

Epidemiology
- 10 cases per 100,000 people
- >90% neurogenic
- <1% arterial

Pathogenesis
- Arterial: Emboli from aneurysm or subclavian artery stenosis
- Venous: Thrombosis or other subclavian vein obstruction

Risk Factors
- Cervical rib found in <1% of the population (70% seen in women); most are asymptomatic
- Most cervical ribs cause neurogenic thoracic outlet syndrome (TOS)

Clinical Features
- Hand and forearm symptoms greater than neck and shoulder symptoms

Natural History
- May develop spontaneously
- Venous TOS may develop after excessive use of the upper limb

Diagnosis

Differential diagnosis
- Raynaud's phenomenon
- Cervical radiculopathy
- Brachial plexopathy
- Neurogenic TOS
- Posterior shoulder girdle myofascial pain syndrome
- Sympathetic response

History
- Neck trauma
- Limb pain, paresthesias, shoulder/arm/hand weakness, neck pain, and occipital headaches, as for neurogenic TOS
- Arterial: pallor, coldness, paresthesias
- Venous: arm swelling, cyanosis, aching pain, paresthesias worst in hand/fingers
- May have symptoms of Raynaud's phenomenon

Examination
- Arterial: digital ischemia, pallor, coldness
- Venous: arm swelling and cyanosis, which may be worst distally
- Nerve tension tests and scalene palpation, as for neurogenic TOS

Testing
- Cervical plain films to evaluate for cervical rib
- Duplex ultrasound testing to evaluate vasculature
- Arteriography for vascular surgery planning

Pitfalls
- Adson's Test is of little to no clinical value in any type of TOS

Red flags
- Raynaud's phenomenon may cause confusion with arterial TOS

Treatment

Medical
- Little evidence to support a specific treatment

Exercise
- None indicated

Modalities
- None indicated

Injection
- None indicated

Surgical
- First cervical rib resection
- Surgical repair of artery if abnormalities seen

Consults
- Vascular surgery

Complications of treatment
- Surgery: incisional pain, pneumothorax, intercostobrachial neuralgia, wound infection, wound hematoma

Prognosis
- Unknown
- Rare surgery
- May require several opinions and consults from TOS experts

Helpful Hint
- Differentiate between arterial and venous causes, rather than lumping the two together as "vascular TOS"

Suggested Readings
Povlsen B, Belzberg A, Hansson T, et al. *Treatment for thoracic outlet syndrome* (Review). The Cochrane Collaboration. Indianapolis, IN: J Wiley & Sons; 2010.

Sanders RJ, Hammond SL, Rao NM. Diagnosis of thoracic outlet syndrome. *J Vascular Surg.* 2007;46(3):601–604.

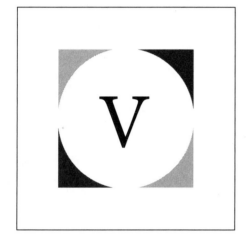

Motor Neuron
Diseases

Amyotrophic Lateral Sclerosis

Cynthia L. Bodkin MD

Description

Amyotrophic lateral sclerosis (ALS) is a progressive neurodegenerative disorder affecting the motor neurons in the brain and spinal cord.

Etiology/Types

- Approximately 10% is genetic
- 90% sporadic with unknown cause
- Progressive bulbar palsy—primarily affects bulbar muscles
- Progressive muscular atrophy—only lower motor neuron findings
- Primary lateral sclerosis—only upper motor neuron findings

Epidemiology

- Prevalence estimated 6 per 100,000
- Incidence 2 per 100,000
- White population more commonly affected
- Male-to-female ratio of 1.5:1
- Age of onset is most often between 40 and 70 years, but can be any age

Pathogenesis

- Unknown in majority of cases
- Roughly 10% to 15% of the genetic cases are from superoxide dismutase 1 mutation
- Other known genes TDP-43 (TAR DNA-binding protein-43), FUS (fused in sarcoma/translated in liposarcoma) gene, and valosin-containing protein

Risk Factors

- Service in United States military
- Deployed in Gulf War

Clinical Features

- Painless progressive weakness starts in one area and spreads to rest of body
- Lower motor neuron signs, such as fasciculations and atrophy
- Upper motor neuron (corticospinal track) signs, such as spasticity, brisk reflexes, and Babinski reflex
- Pseudobulbar affect
- Frontotemporal dementia

Natural History

- Progressive weakness of skeletal muscles, including respiratory muscles, leading to respiratory failure

Diagnosis

Differential diagnosis

- Cervical spondylosis
- Multifocal motor neuropathy with conduction block
- Myasthenia gravis
- Spinal muscular atrophy

History

- Progressive painless weakness
- Twitching or fasciculations
- Cramps
- Muscle atrophy or wasting
- Shortness of breath
- Dysarthria
- Dysphagia
- Falls

Examination

- Muscle weakness
- Atrophy
- Spasticity
- Brisk reflexes
- Abnormal reflexes
- Fasciculations
- Sensory generally preserved

Testing

- Nerve conduction studies (NCS)—decreased motor amplitudes with normal sensory responses
- EMG—fibrillation and fasciculation potentials with large complex motor unit potentials
- Magnetic resonance imaging (MRI) brain and spine—rule out other causes
- Gene testing if family history exists
- Rapid plasma reagin (RPR)—rule out syphilis
- B12
- HIV
- Anti-GM1 antibodies in pure lower motor neuron disease
- Anti-acetylcholine receptor antibodies
- Anti-muscle specific kinase (MuSK) antibodies
- Hexosaminidase A
- Lyme disease

Pitfalls
- Delayed diagnosis

Red flags
- Gynecomastia suggests Kennedy's disease

Treatment

Medical
- Riluzole
- Dextromethorphan/quinidine for pseudobulbar affect
- Supportive
- Bilevel positive airway pressure
- Feeding tube

Exercises
- Stretching
- Range of motion
- Avoid aggressive physical therapy or strengthening

Modalities
- Active and/or passive range of motion

Surgical
- Tracheostomy and ventilation depending on patient's wishes:
  - Percutaneous endoscopic gastrostomy tube placement depending on patient's wishes

Consults
- Neurology
- Physical medicine and rehabilitation
- Pulmonary
- Speech Pathology
- Physical Therapy
- Occupational Therapy
- Dietitian

Complications of treatment
- Nausea and elevated liver function test from riluzole
- Dextromethorphan/quinidine—arrhythmias in patients with prolonged QT interval

Prognosis
- Progressive weakness until completely paralyzed or until respiratory failure
- Mean survival 2 to 5 years after onset of weakness

Helpful Hints
- Quality of life main treatment goal
- Beware of painless weakness

Suggested Readings

Amato AA, Russell JA. *Neuromuscular disorders* (pp. viii, 775). New York: McGraw-Hill Medical; 2008.

Brown WF, Bolton CF, Aminoff MJ. *Neuromuscular Function and Disease: Basic, Clinical, and Electrodiagnostic Aspects.* 1st ed. 2 volumes, (pp. xxiii, 1948). Philadelphia, PA: Saunders; 2002.

V: Motor Neuron Diseases

Hereditary Spastic Paraplegia

Gabriel Smith MD ■ Nathan D. Prahlow MD

Description

A genetic, neurodegenerative disorder characterized by progressive spasticity and weakness of the lower limbs.

Etiology/Types

- Hereditary Spastic Paraplegia (HSP) is a hereditary condition
- Autosomal dominant, autosomal recessive and X-linked recessive inheritance patterns
- Uncomplicated (pure) HSP
- Complicated HSP: Pure HSP + other neurologic dysfunction

Epidemiology

- Prevalence is 3 to 10 cases per 100,000
- Male-to-female ratio of 1:2
- Age ranging from infancy to 70 years

Pathogenesis

- Inheritance of mutations results in retrograde degeneration of the longest nerve fibers in the corticospinal tracts and dorsal columns

Risk Factors

- Family history of HSP

Clinical Features

- Classically, pure HSP is characterized by subtle development of leg stiffness, weakness, and increased tone with spared sensation
- Complicated HSP is comprised of pure HSP and additional neurologic and cognitive deficits, including ataxia, mental retardation, peripheral neuropathy, and epilepsy
- Severity of disease is highly variable

Natural History

- Inherited mutations lead to protein dysfunction in various intracellular sites throughout nerve cells of the corticospinal tracts and dorsal columns
- Impaired membrane trafficking and axonal transport lead to neurodegeneration
- Patients experience gradual stiffening and weakness in the lower limbs with variable loss of function

Diagnosis

Differential diagnosis

- Cerebral palsy
- Multiple sclerosis
- Krabbe disease
- HIV/AIDS
- Vitamin deficiency (B12 and E)
- Wilson's disease

History

- Family history of HSP
- Weakness and spasticity of legs develops over months
- Walking impairment due to foot drop
- Urinary urgency
- Patients with complicated HSP demonstrate deterioration in cognitive function and other neurologic functioning

Examination

- Lower extremity muscle weakness, increased tone, and increased deep tendon reflexes
- Upper extremity muscle tone and strength are normal
- Foot drop on gait examination

Testing

- *SPG4* and *SPG3A* (mutated genetic loci)
- Venereal Disease Research Laboratory test—rule out syphilis
- HIV antibody
- Lumbar puncture—evaluate for multiple sclerosis
- Vitamins B12 and E
- Serum copper and ceruloplasmin
- Galactosylceramide beta-galactosidase
- EMG
- Magnetic resonance imaging (MRI)—rule out spine pathology

Pitfalls

- Delayed diagnosis

Red flags

- Development of further neurologic or cognitive decline in HSP patients

Treatment

Medical
- Baclofen (taken orally or intrathecally)
- Tizanadine and dantrolene also decrease spasticity
- Oxybutynin for urinary urgency
- Selective serotonin reuptake inhibitors (SSRIs) for depression due to loss of function

Exercises
- Physical therapy—stretching, strengthening, and walking exercises

Modalities
- Heat for muscle pain

Injection
- Botulinum toxin injections for spasticity

Surgical
- None

Consults
- Neurology
- Physical and occupational therapy
- Physical medicine and rehabilitation

Complications of treatment
- Antispasticity medications may make walking more difficult because stiffness and spasticity may actually help compensate for weakness

Prognosis
- HSP is quite heterogeneous with variable prognoses
- In general, uncomplicated HSP is not associated with increased mortality
- Complicated HSP is associated with greater morbidity and mortality due to additional neurocognitive deficits

Helpful Hint
- Obtaining a thorough family history is very important in making a correct diagnosis

Suggested Readings
Fink J. Advances in the hereditary spastic paraplegias. *Exp Neurol.* 2003;184:106–110.

Salinas S, et al. Hereditary spastic paraplegia: Clinical features and pathogenetic mechanisms. *Lancet Neurol.* 2008;7(12):1127–1138.

V: Motor Neuron Diseases

Poliomyelitis

Gabriel Smith MD ■ Nathan D. Prahlow MD

Description
A viral disease affecting the anterior horn motor neurons of the spinal cord and the nerve cells within the bulbar region of the brainstem, leading to flaccid weakness or paralysis.

Etiology/Types
- Poliomyelitis is caused by poliovirus, a member of the enterovirus group
- Spread is mainly by fecal-oral route
- Types include subclinical poliomyelitis, nonparalytic poliomyelitis, and paralytic poliomyelitis; may also be divided by affected location: spinal poliomyelitis, bulbar poliomyelitis, and bulbospinal poliomyelitis

Epidemiology
- Very rare (<1500 cases worldwide)
- Male-to-female ratio of 1:1
- Most common in children <5 years old:
  - Bulbospinal poliomyelitis accounts for 19% of cases
  - Bulbar poliomyelitis accounts for 2% of cases

Pathogenesis
- Infection with poliovirus

Risk Factors
- Lack of immunization
- Age <5 years
- Travel to endemic area

Clinical Features
- Most infections with poliovirus are asymptomatic (subclinical poliomyelitis)
- Fever, malaise, sore throat, anorexia, and headache (nonparalytic poliomyelitis)
- Severe myalgias followed by flaccid, asymmetric proximal weakness in legs (most common), arms or muscles of the trunk
- Irreversible paralysis, exceedingly dangerous when muscles of respiration are involved

Natural History
- Poliovirus enters nervous system via axonal transport through peripheral nerves, or by crossing the blood–brain barrier
- Incubation of 3 to 6 days
- Progressive inflammation of nerves leads to cell death and can result in paralysis if damage is sufficient (>90% neuronal cell death)

Diagnosis

Differential diagnosis
- Guillain-Barré syndrome
- West Nile virus
- Viral myositis

History
- Recent travel to endemic area
- Unavailability (or refusal) of polio vaccine
- Poor hygiene
- Fever, myalgias
- Asymmetric, proximal weakness

Examination

Minor Illness
- Nausea/vomiting
- Fever, abdominal pain

Major Illness
- Exam consistent with aseptic meningitis
- Profound asymmetric weakness/paralysis
- Contractures

Testing
- Cerebrospinal fluid (pressure/cell count/protein)
- Complete blood count
- EMG
- Throat, stool, blood samples for poliovirus
- Polymerase chain reaction to distinguish wild-type poliovirus from vaccine strains

Pitfalls
- Delayed diagnosis
- Vaccination of immunocompromised patients may lead to contraction of disease
- Poor compliance with vaccination, and difficulty with maintaining accurate records in endemic regions

Red flags
- Respiratory distress/failure
- Muscle weakness or paralysis decades following polio illness (post-polio syndrome)

Treatment

Medical
- Supportive treatment as there is no cure
- Treatment is aimed at prevention
- Vaccination with injected polio vaccine (*inactive*) or oral polio vaccine (*active*, used mainly in endemic regions)

Exercises
- Physical therapy—passive range of motion and splinting help prevent contracture
- Frequent repositioning in paralyzed patients
- Speech therapy to prevent aspiration in patients with cranial nerve involvement

Modalities
- Heat for muscle pain

Injection
- Injectable polio vaccine (IPV) is injectable form of inactivated vaccine

Surgical
- Release of contractures

Consults
- Neurology
- Infectious disease
- Orthopedic surgery
- Pulmonology
- Physical medicine and rehabilitation

Complications of treatment
- Much higher rate of vaccine-induced polio in immunocompromised patients

Prognosis
- Infection is asymptomatic in most cases
- Patients with nonparalytic polio recover fully
- About 5% patients with paralytic polio die from respiratory failure
- Post-polio syndrome may occur 20 to 40 years following bout with paralytic polio (prognosis is good)

Helpful Hints
- Polio is nearly eradicated
- Goal is prevention with vaccination
- Be aware of post-polio syndrome in patients with history of paralytic polio

Suggested Reading
Cohen JI. Enteroviruses and reoviruses. *Harrison's Principles of Internal Medicine.* 17th ed. New York: McGraw Hill; 2008.

V: Motor Neuron Diseases

Post-Polio Syndrome

Shangming Zhang MD FAAPMR

Description

Post-poliomyelitis syndrome (PPS) is a complex of late onset of neuromuscular symptoms that occurs decades after a patient has recovered from the acute polio infection. The common symptoms include fatigue, new muscle weakness or atrophy, and musculoskeletal pain. Patients also frequently complain of difficulties with walking and stair-climbing.

Etiology/Types

- Unclear. The most accepted hypothesis is that excess metabolic demand on remaining motor neurons leads to their eventual deterioration

Epidemiology

- 29% to 64% of polio survivors
- 200,000 to 640,000 PPS cases in the United States
- 12 to 20 million worldwide
- Onset of PPS approximately 30 years after acute polio
- Affects women more than men

Pathogenesis

The precise cause of PPS remains unclear. Several hypotheses have been proposed as follows:

- Remaining healthy motor neurons cannot maintain new sprouts due to denervation exceeding reinnervation
- Chronic inflammation or cellular immunity-mediated process
- Reactivation of persistent latent viruses causes motor neuronal loss
- Aging: the interval between acute polio and PPS is a risk factor for PPS

Risk Factors

- Severe residual weakness
- Early bulbar respiratory difficulty in the acute phase
- Aging

Clinical Features

- Muscle or joint pain
- Fatigue
- Muscle weakness and atrophy
- Poor endurance

- Sleep apnea
- Swallowing or breathing problems

Natural History

- Slowly progressive with period of stability of 3 to 10 years

Diagnosis

Differential diagnosis

- Peripheral polyneuropathy
- Myopathy
- Multilevel radiculopathy
- West Nile virus infection
- Amyotrophic lateral sclerosis
- Multiple sclerosis
- Myasthenia gravis

History

- Confirmed history of acute paralytic polio with residual muscle weakness and atrophy
- A period of partial or complete functional recovery after acute polio, followed by interval of stable neurologic function for at least 15 years
- Fatigue
- New onset or increased muscle weakness and atrophy
- Muscle and or joint pain
- Symptoms at least 1 year

Examination

- Progressive weakness in previously weak muscle groups or new weakness in previously clinically unaffected muscle groups
- Weakness
- Deep tendon reflexes absent
- Sensation intact
- Electromyographic evidence of denervation

Pitfalls

- Misdiagnosis for any of the conditions described in the differential diagnosis

Red flags

- Occult fractures—may be overlooked in case of muscle pain

Treatment

Medical
- Lamotrigine, bromocriptine, and pyridostigmine reported to improve fatigue
- Modafinil and corticosteroids ineffective
- IVIG 2 g/kg over 2 to 5 days in refractory cases

Exercise
- Rehabilitation management is the mainstay of treatment
- Submaximal aerobic training and low-intensity muscular strengthening
- Aquatic therapy has a positive impact on pain and muscle function

Modalities
- Transcutaneous electrical nerve stimulation (TENS) unit, heat, ice can be used to manage pain

Injections
- Nerve blocks effective to relieve pain

Surgical
- Joint deformities, contractures, and leg length discrepancy may require surgery

Consults
- Interventional pain management for nerve blocks

Complications of treatment
- Fractures
- Falls
- Upper extremity entrapment neuropathy

Prognosis
- Slowly progressive with period of stability of 3 to 10 years

Helpful Hints
- PPS is essentially a diagnosis of exclusion made in polio survivors
- Due to high-risk group for fall and fracture, bone density assessment, review of fall risk, and therapeutic intervention should be considered for all PPS patients
- Pain is the most common complaint in >90% of cases. Most frequently reported pain sites are shoulders, lower back, legs, and hips

Suggested Reading
Gonzalez H, Olsson T, Borg K. Management of postpolio syndrome. *Lancet Neurol.* 2010;9:634–642.

V: Motor Neuron Diseases

Primary Lateral Sclerosis

Cynthia L Bodkin MD

Description
Primary lateral sclerosis (PLS) is a progressive neurodegenerative disorder affecting the upper motor neurons in the brain and spinal cord.

Etiology/Types
- Unknown

Epidemiology
- Unclear
- Approximately 0.5% of patients with amyotrophic lateral sclerosis (ALS)
- Male-to-female estimated ratio of 1:1
- Age of onset is similar to ALS

Pathogenesis
- Unknown

Risk Factors
- None known

Clinical Features
- Progressive stiffness and weakness, usually starting in the lower extremities then spreading to rest of the body
- Upper motor neuron (corticospinal track) signs, such as spasticity, brisk reflexes, and Babinski reflex
- Can have pain due to spasticity

Natural History
- Progressive spasticity and weakness of skeletal muscles

Diagnosis

Differential diagnosis
- Cervical spondylosis
- Hereditary spastic paraparesis
- Progressive multiple sclerosis
- ALS
- B12 deficiency

History
- Progressive spasticity and weakness
- Pain from spasticity

- Spastic dysarthria
- Falls

Examination
- Muscle weakness
- Spasticity
- Brisk reflexes
- Abnormal reflexes

Testing
- Nerve conduction studies (NCS)—normal
- Magnetic resonance imaging (MRI) of brain and spine—rule out other causes
- Rapid plasma reagin (RPR)—rule out syphilis
- B12
- HIV
- Cerebrospinal fluid—multiple sclerosis panel
- Lyme disease
- Gene testing for hereditary spastic paraparesis

Pitfalls
- Delayed diagnosis

Red flags
- Family history
- Visual symptoms

Treatment

Medical
- Baclofen
- Tizanidine
- Benzodiazepines
- Supportive
- Bilevel positive airway pressure
- Feeding tube

Exercises
- Stretching
- Range of motion

Modalities
- Active and/or passive range of motion
- Massage
- Pool therapy

Injection
- Botulism toxin for spasticity management

Surgical

- Tracheostomy and ventilation depending on patient's wishes
  - Percutaneous endoscopic gastrostomy tube placement depending on patient's wishes
- Baclofen pump for spasticity management

Consults

- Neurology
- Physical medicine and rehabilitation
- Pulmonary
- Speech pathology
- Physical and occupational therapist
- Dietitian

Complications of treatment

- Nausea and elevated liver function test from medications

- Sedation
- Confusion

Prognosis

- Progressive weakness and stiffness until completely paralyzed or until respiratory failure
- Average disease duration is 20 years
- Some "PLS" patients may later develop lower motor neuron findings

Helpful Hint

- Quality of life main treatment goal

Suggested Readings

Amato AA, Russell JA. *Neuromuscular Disorders* (pp. viii, 775). New York: McGraw-Hill Medical; 2008.

Brown WF, Bolton CF, Aminoff MJ. *Neuromuscular Function and Disease : Basic, Clinical, and Electrodiagnostic Aspects.* 1st ed. 2 volumes (pp. xxiii, 1948). Philadelphia, PA: Saunders; 2002.

V: Motor Neuron Diseases

Progressive Bulbar Palsy

Cynthia L. Bodkin MD

Description

Progressive bulbar palsy is a progressive neurodegenerative disorder affecting the lower motor neurons to the facial muscles involved in swallowing, chewing, and speaking.

Etiology/Types

- Unknown

Epidemiology

- Unclear
- Approximately 25% of patients with amyotrophic lateral sclerosis present with bulbar symptoms
- Age of onset usually between 50 and 70 years, but can be seen in any age

Pathogenesis

- Majority unknown
- SOD1 mutation

Risk Factors

- Family history

Clinical Features

- Progressive dysphagia and dysarthria
- Choking
- Pneumonia
- Emotional liability

Natural History

- Progressive weakness of bulbar muscles leading to inability to speak or swallow

Diagnosis

Differential diagnosis

- Myasthenia gravis
- Brain stem stroke
- Ocularpharyngeal muscular dystrophy

History

- Choking
- Slurred speech

- Difficulty chewing
- Drooling

Examination

- Bulbar muscle weakness
- Fasciculations in bulbar muscles
- Less prominent arm and leg weakness with upper and lower motor neuron findings
- Abnormal reflexes

Testing

- Nerve conduction studies (NCS)—fasciculation and fibrillation potentials with large complex motor unit potentials diffusely
- Magnetic resonance imaging (MRI) of brain and spine—rule out other causes
- HIV
- Lyme disease
- Acetylcholine receptor antibodies

Pitfalls

- Delayed diagnosis

Red flags

- Visual symptoms such as double vision
- Eye movement abnormalities

Treatment

Medical

- Anticholinergic medication for drooling
- Supportive
- Bilevel positive airway pressure
- Feeding tube

Exercises

- Stretching and range of motion for limb symptoms

Injection

- Botulism toxin to the parotid gland for saliva management

Surgical

- Tracheostomy and ventilation depending on patient's wishes
  - Percutaneous endoscopic gastrostomy tube placement depending on patient's wishes

Consults
- Neurology
- Physical medicine and rehabilitation
- Pulmonary
- Speech pathology
- Physical and occupational therapist
- Dietitian

Complications of treatment
- Nausea and elevated liver function test from medications
- Sedation
- Confusion
- Dry mouth
- Urinary retention

Prognosis
- Progressive weakness of bulbar muscles until respiratory failure from pneumonia
- Survival 1 to 3 years

Helpful Hint
- Quality of life main treatment goal

Suggested Readings
Amato AA, Russell JA. *Neuromuscular Disorders* (p. viii, 775). New York: McGraw-Hill Medical; 2008.

Brown WF, Bolton CF, Aminoff MJ. *Neuromuscular Function and Disease: Basic, Clinical, and Electrodiagnostic Aspects.* 1st ed., 2 volumes (pp. xxiii, 1948). Philadelphia, PA: Saunders; 2002.

Progressive Muscular Atrophy

Cynthia L. Bodkin MD

Description

Progressive muscular atrophy is a progressive neurodegenerative disorder affecting the lower motor neurons only.

Etiology/Types

- Unknown
- Flail arm variant
- Flail leg variant

Epidemiology

- Estimated to be around 4% of amyotrophic lateral sclerosis (ALS) cases
- Males more likely to be affected
- Younger age of onset than typical ALS

Pathogenesis

- Unknown

Risk Factors

- None known

Clinical Features

- Painless progressive weakness starts in one area and spreads to the rest of body
- Lower motor neuron signs such as fasciculations and atrophy

Natural History

- Progressive weakness of skeletal muscles, including respiratory muscles, leading to respiratory failure

Diagnosis

Differential diagnosis

- Multifocal motor neuropathy with conduction block
- Spinal muscular atrophy
- Classic ALS

History

- Progressive painless weakness
- Twitching or fasciculations
- Cramps
- Muscle atrophy or wasting
- Shortness of breath
- Falls

Examination

- Muscle weakness
- Atrophy
- Fasciculations
- Sensation generally preserved

Testing

- Nerve conduction studies (NCS)—decreased motor amplitudes with normal sensory responses
- EMG—fibrillation and fasciculation potentials with large complex motor unit potentials
- Magnetic resonance imaging (MRI) of the brain and spine—rule out other causes
- Anti-GM1 antibodies
- Hexosaminidase A
- Lyme disease

Pitfalls

- Delayed diagnosis

Red flags

- Gynecomastia suggests Kennedy's disease

Treatment

Medical

- Riluzole
- Supportive
- Bilevel positive airway pressure
- Feeding tube

Exercises

- Stretching
- Range of motion
- Avoid aggressive physical therapy or strengthening

Modalities

- Active and/or passive range of motion

Surgical

- Tracheostomy and ventilation depending on patient's choice
- Percutaneous endoscopic gastrostomy tube placement depending on patient's choice

Consults

- Neurology
- Physical medicine and rehabilitation
- Pulmonary
- Speech pathology

- Physical and occupational therapist
- Dietitian

Complications of treatment
- Nausea and elevated liver function test from Riluzole

Prognosis
- Progressive weakness until completely paralyzed or until respiratory failure
- Similar to classic ALS (2–5 years) with possible slightly slower course
- Flail limb variants' 5-year survival ranges from 52% to 64%

Helpful Hints
- Quality of life—main treatment goal
- Beware of painless weakness

Suggested Readings

Amato AA, Russell JA. *Neuromuscular Disorders* (pp. viii, 775). New York: McGraw-Hill Medical; 2008.

Brown WF, Bolton CF, Aminoff MJ. *Neuromuscular Function and Disease: Basic, Clinical, and Electrodiagnostic Aspects.* 1st ed., 2 volumes (pp. xxiii, 1948). Philadelphia, PA: Saunders; 2002.

Wijesekera LC, Mathers S, Talman P, Galtrey C, et al. Natural history and clinical features of the flail arm and flail leg ALS variants. *Neurology.* 2009;72(12):1084–1094.

V: Motor Neuron Diseases

Spinal and Bulbar Muscular Atrophy (Kennedy's Disease)

Nathan D. Prahlow MD

Description

A progressive, X-linked, degenerative motor neuron disease, characterized by asymmetric weakness in the hip and shoulder girdle musculature and associated muscle cramping, atrophy, and fasciculations. Speech and swallowing difficulties develop as the disease progresses.

Etiology/Types

- Almost exclusively affects males
- Female carriers, because of lyonization, may have mild muscle cramps and weakness, fasciculations, and elevated creatine kinase levels

Epidemiology

- X-linked recessive
- Prevalence of 3.3 per 100,000, but geographically variable, with a prevalence of 13 per 85,000 near Vaasa, Finland

Pathogenesis

- Expansion of the CAG trinucleotide repeat in the androgen receptor gene on chromosome Xq11-12
- Affected subjects typically have repeat counts greater than 40; normal individuals have 11–33 repeats
- Loss of anterior horn cells in the brainstem and spinal cord

Risk Factors

- Mother as a carrier of the abnormality

Clinical Features

- Weakness and wasting of limb, bulbar, and facial muscles, in an asymmetric distribution
- Proximal flaccid weakness (initially lower limbs), which progresses over time
- Bilateral Dupuytren's contractures may be present
- Dysarthria and dysphagia are common; respiratory difficulties may arise
- Postural tremor and easy fatigability may be seen

- Endocrine abnormalities, including gynacomastia, reduced fertility rate, azoospermia, oligospermia, and diabetes
- One-third of patients develop inguinal hernias
- The risk of androgenic alopecia is reduced

Natural History

- Age of onset ranges between 20 and 60 years
- Median age to require a handrail to ascend stairs is 49 years
- Median age requiring use of a cane for ambulation is 59 years
- Median age requiring wheelchair for mobility is 61 years
- There may be a significant variability within affected families for age of onset, rate of progression, and severity of disease
- Severity ranges from asymptomatic (elevated creatine kinase only), to severe muscle disease with bulbar involvement requiring mechanical ventilation

Diagnosis

Differential diagnosis

- Amyotrophic lateral sclerosis
- Primary lateral sclerosis
- Adult-onset spinal muscular atrophy
- Various muscular dystrophies
- Multifocal motor neuropathy
- Mitochondrial disorders

History

- Family history
- Physical changes as described above

Examination

- Examine for atrophy, weakness, bulbar abnormalities

Testing

- Serum creatine kinase may be mildly elevated; may be detectable prior to other disease findings

- EMG findings: Decreased compound muscle action potentials, sensory nerve action potentials, and conduction velocities are present, with upper limb abnormalities typically greater than lower limb
- Scrotal skin biopsy shows high degree of nuclear accumulation of mutant androgen receptor protein
- Genetic testing, including demonstration of the expansion of the CAG repeat in the androgen receptor gene, is the gold standard

Pitfalls
- Variability of disease within known affected families may confound the examiner

Red flags
- Severe bulbar symptoms require earlier respiratory intervention

Treatment

Medical
- Symptomatic treatment only
- Research into androgen deprivation is ongoing

Exercise
- Maintenance of range of motion
- No specific recommendations exist, but avoidance of strenuous exercise may be appropriate

Modalities
- Symptomatic treatment, as needed
- For significant respiratory dysfunction, noninvasive positive pressure ventilation may be indicated

Surgical
- Generally none indicated
- Percutaneous endoscopic gastrostomy tube placement might be needed in cases of severe dysphagia (has never been reported)

Consults
- Neurology
- Medical Genetics

Complications of treatment
- Side effects of any medication or intervention attempted

Prognosis
- One of the best prognoses and survival rates of motor neuron diseases
- Some affected males remain asymptomatic for their entire lives
- Disease progression is generally slow; life expectancy is normal or only minimally reduced
- Pneumonia and respiratory failure are common causes of death

Helpful Hint
- The greater the number of CAG repeats, the earlier the onset of symptoms

Suggested Readings
Finsterer J. Bulbar and spinal muscular atrophy (Kennedy's disease): A review. *Eur J Neurol.* 2009;16:556–561.
Finsterer J. Perspectives of Kennedy's disease. *J Neurolog Sci.* 2010;298:1–10.

V: Motor Neuron Diseases

Spinal Muscular Atrophy

Shangming Zhang MD FAAPMR

Description

Spinal muscular atrophy (SMA) is the second most common autosomal-recessive neuromuscular disorder. It is characterized by progressive symmetric muscle weakness due to degeneration and loss of lower motor neurons (anterior horn cells in the spinal cord and cranial nerve nuclei).

Etiology/Types

- Due to mutations in survival motor neuron (SMN) gene
- Acute infantile (SMA type I or Werdnig-Hoffmann disease): onset from birth to 6 months
- Chronic infantile (SMA II): onset between 6 and 12 months
- Chronic juvenile (SMA III or Kugelberg-Welander disease): onset after 12 months
- Adult onset (SMA IV): onset of symptoms during early adulthood with more favorable prognosis

Epidemiology

- Estimated incidence of approximately 1 in 10,000 to 15,000 live births with a genetic carrier frequency of 1 of 50 to 80

Pathogenesis

- Thought to be caused by progressive degeneration and loss of the anterior horn cells in the spinal cord due to mutation, deletion, or rearrangement of SMN genes, which are essential for early pre-mRNA splicing

Risk Factors

- Family history
- Male gender

Clinical Features

- Type I SMA (Werdnig-Hoffmann disease): floppy baby/hypotonia, difficulty feeding, weak cry, failure to reach milestones, absent muscle stretch reflexes, frog-legged position, tongue fasciculations, extraocular and sphincter muscles spared
- Type II SMA: floppy baby/hypotonia, slowly progressive limb weakness, upper greater than lower, absent muscle stretch reflexes, kyphoscoliosis, independent sitting, standing, and walking with assistive devices
- Type III SMA (Kugelberg-Welander disease): symmetric proximal weakness, independent standing and walking but trouble with going up and down stairs, with or without positive Gowers' sign, calf pseudohypertrophy, and normal intelligence
- Type IV SMA: benign, similar to type III

Natural History

- Anterior horn motor neuron degeneration and death
- Peripheral denervation, muscular weakness, atrophy, and pain
- Respiratory failure and death in severe cases

Diagnosis

Differential diagnosis

- Becker muscular dystrophy
- Amyotrophic lateral sclerosis
- Congenital myopathies
- Myasthenia gravis
- Disorders of carpotonia
- Disorders of carbohydrate metabolism
- Botulism
- Acid maltase deficiency
- Primary lateral sclerosis

History

- Type I with poor sucking, difficulty swallowing, frequent respiratory infections and failures
- Type II with developmental motor delay
- Type III with slowly progressive proximal weakness, the pelvic girdle being more affected than the shoulder girdle
- Type IV symptomatic in the mid-thirties

Examination

- Muscle atrophy
- Flaccid weakness
- Fasciculations
- Hypotonia and wasting
- Decreased or absent deep tendon reflexes
- Sensory examination normal
- Normal sensory nerve action potential (SNAP)
- Abnormal needle EMG
- Molecular genetic testing confirmatory
- Increased creatine phosphokinase level
- Electrocardiogram normal

Pitfalls
- Delayed diagnosis
- Genetic counseling and prenatal diagnosis should be offered to all families with SMA

Red flags
- Pulmonary infection and failure
- As symptoms progress, it is unsafe for patients with SMA to drive or operate other machinery
- Increased risk of falls due to weakness in lower extremities

Treatment

Medical
- Supportive
- Knee-ankle-foot orthoses
- Well-fitted wheelchair to prevent spinal deformities and joint contractures

Exercise
- Non–fatigue causing exercise

Modalities
- Transcutaneous electrical nerve stimulation may help symptomatic relief of pain

Surgical
- Spinal deformity correction and early orthopedic intervention if indicated
- Noninvasive ventilation and percutaneous gastrostomy to improve quality of life

Consults
- Physical medicine and rehabilitation
- Spine and orthopedic surgery for deformities
- Gastroenterology
- Pulmonology
- Dietary or nutrition

Complications of treatment
- Exercise-caused pain or fatigue
- Infection from surgical intervention

Prognosis
- Children with SMA type I usually die from respiratory failure within the first 2 years
- The lifespan of patients with SMA type II varies from 2 years to the third decade of life
- Many patients with SMA type III have a normal life expectancy
- Patients with SMA type IV have a normal life expectancy

Helpful Hints
- Facial muscles affected least
- Extraocular muscles, bowel, and bladder spared
- Sensation normal
- Antibiotic treatment not affecting survival in SMA type I

Suggested Reading
Prior T. Spinal muscular atrophy: Newborn and carrier screening. *Obstet Gynecol Clin N Am.* 2010;37:23–36.

V: Motor Neuron Diseases

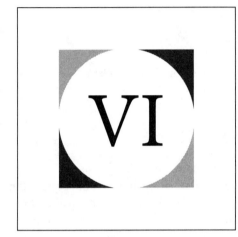

Muscle Diseases

Becker Muscular Dystrophy

Matthew Axtman DO

Description

Becker muscular dystrophy is an inherited disorder of slowly progressive weakening of proximal limb and pelvic muscles caused by a mutation of the dystrophin gene.

Etiology/Types

- X-linked recessive

Epidemiology

- Incidence is 1 per 30,000 male births
- Females are carriers of the mutated dystrophin gene

Pathogenesis

- Mutation of the dystrophin gene, causing a defect in the dystrophin protein
- The dystrophin gene is located on the short arm of chromosome 21 (Xp21)

Risk Factors

- A positive family history of Becker muscular dystrophy

Clinical Features

- Difficulty with ambulation and mobility
- Muscle weakness and symptoms usually develop around the age of 11 years but can occur earlier or later
- Patients usually remain ambulatory until their late twenties

Natural History

- Muscle atrophy in proximal muscles due to dystrophin mutation
- Proliferation of adipose and connective tissue within the muscles
- Affects skeletal and smooth muscles, therefore both voluntary and cardiac tissues involved

Diagnosis

Differential diagnosis

- Duchenne muscular dystrophy
- Congenital muscular dystrophy
- Facioscapulohumeral dystrophy
- Limb-girdle muscular dystrophy
- Emery-Dreifuss muscular dystrophy
- Spinal muscular atrophy

History

- Progressive difficulty with walking, running, jumping, climbing stairs
- Frequent falls
- Loss of balance
- Difficulty breathing
- Mild learning and cognitive problems
- Fatigue

Examination

- Calf pseudohypertrophy
- Muscle atrophy
- Symmetrical proximal muscle weakness
- Gowers Sign—a maneuver in which the patient starts in a 4-point stance on the hands and knees and slowly uses the hands to "walk up" the legs to a standing position. This is due to weak pelvic girdle muscles and proximal hip weakness
- Waddling gait
- Toe walking
- Scoliosis

Testing

- Creatine phosphokinase levels may be elevated 5 to 100 times normal levels, but levels decrease as muscle mass decreases
- Muscle biopsy demonstrates variation of muscles' sizes and proliferation of adipose or connective tissue
- Polymerase chain reaction
- Genetic testing for dystrophin abnormalities
- Ultrasonography shows increased echogenicity in affected muscles
- 75% of patients show echocardiogram abnormalities of right ventricular strain, tall R waves, deep Q waves, and inverted T waves
- EMG shows a myopathic pattern of decreased amplitude, polyphasic, short duration motor-unit action potentials

Pitfalls

- Not evaluating cardiac status—cardiac tissue may be more affected than skeletal muscles

Red flags
- Dilated cardiomyopathy—mild
- Respiratory infections
- Respiratory failure

Treatment

Medical
- Patient and family education
- Short-term steroid treatment using prednisone has shown temporary increases in strength
- Creatine supplementation has been shown to enhance athletic performance in up to 10% of individuals
- Evaluation for bracing, walkers, and wheelchairs if mobility becomes limited

Exercises
- Encourage moderate activity
- Stretching
- Physical therapy targeting range of motion to prevent the formation of contractures

Modalities
- None

Surgical
- Spinal fusion for scoliosis
- Tendon release for joint contractures

Consults
- Physical medicine and rehabilitation
- Cardiology
- Pulmonology
- Orthopedic surgery for spinal deformities or tendon release
- Genetic counseling

Complications of treatment
- Effects of long-term steroids
- Strenuous activity can cause muscle damage

Prognosis
- There is a high variability of disability in patients—many patients maintain independence with assistive devices
- Early onset of symptoms is associated with more cardiac involvement and earlier difficulty with mobility
- Patients will most likely need the use of a wheelchair or assistive device for mobility
- Life expectancy is into the 5th and 6th decades of life, but can live a normal lifespan

Helpful Hints
- Activity should be limited to moderate intensity due to the possibility of muscle damage with strenuous activity
- Calf pseudohypertophy is due to increased adipose and connective tissue and not due to increased muscle mass
- Cognitive deficiencies are less severe than in Duchenne muscular dystrophy

Suggested Readings
Louis M, Lebacq J, Poortmans JR, Belpaire-Dethiou MC, et al. Beneficial effects of creatine supplementation in dystrophic patients. *Muscle Nerve.* 2003;27(5):604–610.

Markert CD, Ambrosio F, Call JA, Grange RW. Exercise and Duchenne muscular dystrophy: Toward evidence-based exercise prescription. *Muscle Nerve.* 2011;43(4):464–478.

Dermatomyositis

Shangming Zhang MD FAAPMR

Description

Dermatomyositis is an idiopathic inflammatory myopathy manifested by symmetrical proximal weakness, characteristic skin lesions, and strong association with malignancy.

Etiology/Types

- Unknown etiology
- Type 1: primary idiopathic polymyositis; insidious onset; with dysphagia, dysphonia, and moderate-to-severe arthritis
- Type 2: primary idiopathic dermatomyositis; acute onset; with proximal muscle weakness, heliotrope rash with periorbital edema and systematic symptoms, including fatigue, fever, and weight loss
- Type 3: dermatomyositis or polymyositis; associated with malignancy; seen in males > 40 years old; prognosis poor
- Type 4: childhood dermatomyositis or polymyositis; more disabling due to severe joint contracture; rapidly progressive weakness
- Type 5: dermatomyositis or polymyositis overlapping with collagen vascular disease

Epidemiology

- Estimated prevalence 5.5 in 100,000 people

Pathogenesis

- Activation and deposition of complement causes lysis of endomysial capillaries and muscle ischemia

Risk Factors

- Male-to-female ratio 2:1
- Two peak ages of onset: 5 to 10 years; 50 years

Clinical Features

- Generalized fatigue
- Symmetric proximal weakness
- Characteristic skin lesions:
  - Gottron's papules—erythematous scaly coating at dorsal finger joints
  - Heliotrope rash—violaceous coloration on upper eyelids
  - Shawl sign—erythematous area in a "V" over the upper back or chest
- Dysphagia
- Abnormal cardiopulmonary findings

Natural History

- Striated muscle inflammation and weakness
- Cutaneous lesions
- Association with malignancy: ovarian, lung, pancreatic, stomach, and colorectal cancers, and non-Hodgkin's lymphoma

Diagnosis

Differential diagnosis

- Polymyositis
- Inclusion body myositis
- Systemic lupus erythematous
- Scleroderma
- Plaque psoriasis
- Sarcoidosis

History

- Difficulty climbing stairs, walking, or rising from a sitting position
- Pruritic rash, scaly scalp, or diffuse hair loss
- Arthralgia, arthritis
- Difficulty swallowing or speaking

Examination

- Characteristic heliotrope (blue-purple discoloration) rash with periorbital edema
- Proximal muscle weakness with or without tenderness
- Joint swelling
- Diffuse alopecia
- Gottron's papules over bony prominences
- Periungual telangiectases, poikiloderma
- Calcinosis cutis—calcium deposition in skin, seen in juvenile form

Testing

- Elevated creatine kinase, aldolase, lactate dehydrogenase (LDH)
- Positive antinuclear antigen
- Myopathic findings on EMG
- Biopsy: perifascicular atrophy, large nuclei, necrosis

Pitfalls

- Misdiagnosis of skin disease as psoriasis or eczema
- Failure to screen malignancy associated with dermatomyositis
- Delayed initiation of corticosteroid therapy

Red flags
- Presence of malignancy
- Cardiopulmonary involvement

Treatment

Medical
- Oral *corticosteroids* as the mainstay of therapy: prednisone 1 mg/kg/day for 4 to 6 weeks, then taper to avoid relapse
- Immunosuppressive agents as second line: azathioprine or methotrexate
- Intravenous immunoglobulin (IVIg) in severe refractory cases
- Sun protection cream

Exercise
- Encourage range-of-motion and isometric exercises
- No strengthening exercises until inflammation controlled
- Sun avoidance and protective measures in patients with skin lesions

Modalities
- Heat, cold, ultrasound can be tried in patients with contractures

Surgical
- Surgery for resectable malignancy
- Surgical removal of calcinosis

Consults
- Rheumatology
- Dermatology
- Neurology
- Medical and Surgical Oncology
- Cardiology
- Internal Medicine

Complications of treatment
- Side effects of corticosteroids

Prognosis
- Depending on severity of myopathy, coexistence of malignancy, and cardiopulmonary involvement
- 20% cases have spontaneous remission and 5% have rapid progressive course and death

Helpful Hints
- Mandatory screening for malignancy
- Heliotrope rash strongly suggestive of dermatomyositis
- Sun avoidance and protective measures necessary for patients with skin disease

Suggested Reading
Dalakas MC, Hohlfeld R. Polymyositis and dermatomyositis. *Lancet.* 2003;362:971–982.

VI: Muscle Diseases

Duchenne Muscular Dystrophy

Shangming Zhang MD FAAPMR

Description
Duchenne muscular dystrophy (DMD) is an X-linked recessive disorder caused by chronic muscle degeneration due to dystrophin deficiency. DMD is severe, progressive, and the most common muscular dystrophy.

Etiology/Types
- X-linked recessive (Xp 21.2) inherited
- Spontaneous deletions or mutations

Epidemiology
- Most common childhood-onset muscular dystrophy
- Affecting 1 in 3600 to 6000 live male births

Pathogenesis
- Dystrophin protein is essential to the structural stability of myofibers. Dystrophin deficiency associated with DMD results in chronic inflammation and severe muscular degeneration.
- Dystrophin deficiency also leads to cardiomyopathy and possible mental retardation

Risk Factors
- Family history

Clinical Features
- Delayed motor milestones
- Waddling gait and Gower's sign by age 3 to 5 years
- Calf pseudohypertrophy with fatty and fibrous tissue replacement within 1 to 2 years
- Toe walking and clumsy running
- Gower's sign (patient uses hands/arms to "climb" up their body to arise from floor) is due to proximal muscle weakness
- Lumbar lordosis and scoliosis
- Wheelchair bound by 12 years old
- Possible mental retardation
- Extraocular muscles spared

Natural History
- Chronic progressive muscular degeneration
- Weakness, contractures, scoliosis, wheelchair bound, decubitus ulcers, pulmonary complications, and cardiomyopathy to death

Diagnosis

Differential diagnosis
- Becker muscular dystrophy
- Myotonic muscular dystrophy (Steinert's disease)
- Spinal muscular atrophy
- Facioscapulohumeral dystrophy
- Kennedy's disease
- Limb-girdle muscular dystrophy
- Metabolic myopathy

History
- Onset of symptoms in childhood
- Weakness, fatigue, and poor endurance
- Frequent falls, difficulty ascending stairs, or arising from the floor
- Muscle cramps or stiffness
- Focal enlargement of calf muscles
- Lordosis and scoliosis
- Family history

Examination
- Proximal muscle weakness
- Calf enlargement
- Abnormal deep tendon reflexes
- Increased creatine phosphokinase with values up to 50 to 100 times normal
- Abnormal electrocardiogram
- EMG: sensory nerve action potential (SNAP) normal, compound muscle action potential (CMAP) small amplitude, needle exam with myopathic findings
- Muscle biopsy: no dystrophin
- X-ray to evaluate and screen the degree of spine deformities
- Molecular diagnosis

Pitfalls
- Cardiac surveillance to be implemented at the time of diagnosis

Red flags
- Osteoporosis and fractures

Treatment

Medical

- Prednisone 0.75 to 1.5 mg/kg p.o. daily: extension of independent ambulation up to 3 years, delay in development of scoliosis and cardiac and respiratory complications
- H2 blocker to prevent corticosteroids—caused gastritis and ulcer

Exercise

- Gentle sports and activities under supervision
- Daily stretching to delay contractures

Modalities

- Heat, cold, ultrasound may provide relief of contracture-related pain

Surgical

- Scoliosis surgery before vital capacity less than 35%
- Tendon lengthening surgery may prolong ambulation by up to 2 years

Consults

- Orthopedic surgery
- Cardiology
- Pulmonology
- Neurology
- Genetics
- Psychology

Complications of treatment

- Corticosteroids can cause cataracts, diabetes, hypertension, osteoporosis, behavioral changes, and weight gain
- Infection and failures related to surgical intervention

Prognosis

- Onset at age 3 to 5 years
- Wheelchair bound by age of 12 years
- Death by age of 20 years

Helpful Hints

- Corticosteroid treatment has been proved to prolong independent ambulation by up to 3 years, delays development of scoliosis, and improves cardiac and respiratory functions
- Coordinated multidisciplinary care needed

Suggested Readings

Bushby K, Finkel R, Birnkrant DJ, Case LE, et al. Diagnosis and management of Duchenne muscular dystrophy, part 1: Diagnosis, and pharmacological and psychosocial management. *Lancet Neurol.* 2010;9:77–93.

Bushby K, Finkel R, Birnkrant DJ, Case LE, et al. Diagnosis and management of Duchenne muscular dystrophy, part 2: Implementation of multidisciplinary care. *Lancet Neurol.* 2010;9:177–189.

Emery-Dreifuss Muscular Dystrophy

Nathan D. Prahlow MD

Description

- Emery-Dreifuss muscular dystrophy is characterized by early formation of contractures and the presence of cardiac issues. It is the third most common X-linked recessive muscular dystrophy, although autosomal recessive and dominant forms are also seen.

Etiology/Types

- X-linked
- Autosomal dominant: variable features
- Autosomal recessive

Epidemiology

- X-linked: 1 per 100,000 people; the most common form of Emery-Dreifuss muscular dystrophy
- Autosomal dominant: unknown
- Autosomal recessive: very rare

Pathogenesis

- Mutations in the EMD or LMNA genes affect proteins in the nuclear lamina of the cell

Risk Factors

- Family history positive for Emery-Dreifuss muscular dystrophy

Clinical Features

- Early formation of joint contractures
- Muscle wasting in humeroperoneal distribution
- Cardiac conduction defects (bradycardia progressing to complete heart block), with or without cardiomyopathy

Natural History

- Normal birth and early development
- Onset in early childhood/adolescence (<15 years)
- Slow progression
- Rare loss of ambulation
- Cardiac issues may develop before significant weakness
- Cardiac involvement is almost always present by age 30 years

Diagnosis

Differential diagnosis

- Duchenne muscular dystrophy
- Becker muscular dystrophy
- Fascioscapulohumeral dystrophy
- Limb-girdle muscular dystrophies

History

- Upper limb functionality (biceps and triceps)
- Palpitations, syncope

Examination

- Irregular cardiac rhythm
- Presence of contractures
- Marked humeral and peroneal muscle wasting, with relative sparing of deltoid
- Inability to heel-walk due to Achilles contracture and calf atrophy
- May be unable to flex lumbar spine due to contractures
- Mild facial weakness
- Mild hand weakness

Testing

- Genetic testing
- Muscle biopsy: nonspecific myopathic changes
- Electrocardiogram (EKG): low amplitude/absent P waves, variable degree of conduction block, possible evidence of cardiomyopathy
- EMG: myopathic features of low amplitude compound muscle action potential (CMAP) in atrophic muscles
- Serum creatine kinase mildly elevated (<10 times normal)

Pitfalls

- Carriers are at risk for sudden death due to arrhythmia

Red flags

- Cardiac arrhythmias, with or without cardiomyopathy

Treatment

Medical treatment

- Supportive
- May require powered mobility
- Cardiac: annual EKG, Holter monitor, antiplatelet therapy, cardiac transplant

Exercise

- Cardiac precautions necessary

Modalities

- Ankle foot orthoses

Injection
■ None indicated

Surgical
■ Pacemaker or automatic implanted cardiac defibrillator
■ Surgical release of contractures

Consults
■ Cardiology
■ Cardiac surgery
■ Orthopedic surgery
■ Certified Orthotist

Complications of treatment
■ Complications of surgery

Prognosis
■ No effective treatment for the progressive weakness

Helpful Hint
■ Annual cardiac screening of relatives is needed, as carriers are at risk for sudden death due to arrhythmia

Suggested Readings
Helbling-Leclerc A, Bonne G, Schwartz K. Emery-Dreifuss muscular dystrophy. *Eur J Human Genetics.* 2002;10: 157–161.
Zacharias AS, Wagener ME, Warren ST, et al. Emery-Dreifuss muscular dystrophy. *Semin Neurol.* 1999;19(1):67–79.

VI: Muscle Diseases

Fascioscapulohumeral Dystrophy

Matthew Axtman DO

Description

Fascioscapulohumeral dystrophy is a slowly progressive weakening of skeletal muscles, which usually starts in the face, shoulder girdle, and upper arms.

Etiology/Types

- Autosomal dominant in 70% to 90% of patients
- Sporadic mutation in 10% to 30% of individuals

Epidemiology

- Prevalence is 1 in 20,000
- Higher frequency in males

Pathogenesis

- Caused by the deletion of D4Z4 at gene locus 4q35 on chromosome 4

Risk Factors

- A positive family history of fascioscapulohumeral dystrophy

Clinical Features

- Winged scapula
- Facial muscle weakness
- Foot-drop
- Increased lumbar lordosis

Natural History

- Symptoms develop in the 1st to 3rd decade of life
- 90% of patients demonstrate symptoms by the age of 20 years
- Weakness typically begins in the facial muscles and slowly progresses caudally
- Scapular winging is the most common initial symptom

Diagnosis

Differential diagnosis

- Congenital muscular dystrophy
- Amyotrophic lateral sclerosis
- Limb-girdle muscular dystrophy
- Dermatomyositis
- Congenital myopathies

History

- Difficulty whistling
- Difficulty sucking through a straw
- Eye lids remain open while sleeping
- Shoulder weakness
- Winged scapula
- Muscle pain
- Problems with dorsiflexion of the feet

Examination

- Scapular winging
- Weak facial muscles
- Weak tibialis anterior muscle resulting in foot-drop
- Atrophy of the biceps and triceps
- Beevor's sign (movement of the navel toward the head when flexing the neck) due to lower abdominal muscle weakness
- Increased lumbar lordosis due to weak abdominal muscles
- High-frequency sensorineural hearing loss

Testing

- Creatine kinase—elevated
- Muscle biopsy—chronic myopathic changes
- EMG—myopathic potentials

Pitfalls

- Coat's syndrome: retinal vasculopathy with telangiectasia, exudation, and retinal detachment

Red flags

- Vision changes

Treatment

Medical

- Evaluation for bracing, walkers, and wheelchair
- Visual screening

Exercises

- Low-impact aerobic exercises
- Gentle range of motion

Modalities

- Supportive

Surgical

- Scapulothoracic arthrodesis if deltoid function is preserved
- Tendon transfer for foot-drop

Consults

- Physical medicine and rehabilitation
- Neurology
- Ear/nose/throat
- Pulmonology
- Orthopedics
- Audiology
- Ophthalmology
- Genetic counseling

Complications of treatment

- Overuse syndrome
- Pain

Prognosis

- Life expectancy is normal
- 20% of patients may require wheelchair assistance
- Size of the deletion affects prognosis

Helpful Hints

- Extraocular and pharyngeal muscles are spared
- Scapular winging is the most characteristic sign
- Weakness may be asymmetric

Suggested Readings

Pandya S, King WM, Tawil R. Fascioscapulohumeral dystrophy. *Phys Ther.* 2008;88(1):105–113. [Epub 2007 Nov 6].

van der Kooi EL, Vogels OJ, van Asseldonk RJ, et al. Strength training and albuterol in facioscapulohumeral muscular dystrophy. *Neurol.* 2004;24;63(4): 702–708.

Hyperkalemic Periodic Paralysis

Nathan D. Prahlow MD

Description

The periodic paralyses, of which hyperkalemic periodic paralysis (HyperKPP) is a type, are characterized by episodes of flaccid muscle weakness.

Etiology/Types

- Primary (hereditary)
- Secondary (acquired)

Epidemiology

- Autosomal dominant
- 1 in 200,000 people

Pathogenesis

- Mutation in the SCN4A gene, affecting the muscular sodium channel

Risk Factors

- Family history of HyperKPP

Clinical Features

- Attacks of mild-to-severe weakness, worsened by ingestion of potassium-rich foods, strenuous exercise, emotional stress, cold, or medications
- Symptoms may be isolated to a single muscle or widespread
- Usually complete recovery between attacks, but may have stiffness

Natural History

- Onset younger than 10 years
- Frequency and severity of attacks increases gradually as one ages
- Severity decreases after about age 50 years
- Weakness may become permanent

Diagnosis

Differential diagnosis

- Hypokalemic periodic paralysis
- Myotonia congenita
- Paramyotonia congenita
- Myotonic dystrophy
- Schwartz-Jampel syndrome

History

- Symptoms last from minutes up to 4 hours
- Limb, eye, throat, and trunk muscles most involved; respiratory muscles are spared
- Attacks may occur with more frequency before breakfast

Examination

- Myotonia in facial, lingual, and hand muscles
- May have weakness and paresthesias

Testing

- Genetic testing
- Provocative testing with exercise (increases serum potassium) followed by bed rest (immediate decline, followed by increase after 20 minutes of rest)
- EMG: compound muscle action potential (CMAP) amplitude increases after 5 minutes of exercise, and declines within 20 minutes

Pitfalls

- Serum potassium is low after a HyperKPP attack, mimicking hypokalemic periodic paralysis

Red flags

- Avoid potassium, depolarizing muscle relaxants, and cholinesterase inhibitors in general anesthesia

Treatment

Medical

- Genetic counseling
- Ingestion of carbohydrates at onset of symptoms
- Prevent attacks with early awakening and eating of breakfast, frequent carbohydrate-rich meals, avoidance of potassium-rich foods and medications that increase serum potassium, and avoidance of fasting, strenuous exercise, and cold

Exercise

- Mild exercise may help abort an attack

Modalities
- None indicated

Surgical
- None indicated

Consults
- Neurology

Complications of treatment
- Side effects of medications

Prognosis
- Lifespan is not affected

Helpful Hint
- Non-steroidal anti-inflammatory drugs (NSAIDs), heparin, spironolactone, angiotensin converting enzyme (ACE) inhibitors, trimethoprim, and oral/IV potassium may all cause hyperkalemia and induce a secondary HyperKPP

Suggested Readings

Finsterer J. Primary periodic paralyses. *Acta Neurol Scand.* 2008;117:145–158.

Miller TM. Differential diagnosis of myotonic disorders. *Muscle Nerve.* 2008;37:293–299.

Hypokalemic Periodic Paralysis

Nathan D. Prahlow MD

Description
The periodic paralyses, of which hypokalemic periodic paralysis (HypoKPP) is a type, are characterized by episodes of flaccid muscle weakness

Etiology/Types
- Primary (hereditary)
- Secondary (acquired)

Epidemiology
- Autosomal dominant
- 1 in 100,000 people, the most common of the periodic paralyses

Pathogenesis
- Mutation in the CACNA1S gene or SCN4A gene, affecting the voltage-gated sodium channel

Risk Factors
- Family history of HypoKPP

Clinical Features
- Attacks of severe weakness, associated with a drop in serum potassium levels
- Usually complete recovery between attacks, but may have subacute weakness

Natural History
- Onset younger than 20 years
- Frequency and severity of attacks greatest between 15 and 35 years
- Frequency decreases after about age 35 years
- Frequency ranges from a single attack to rare attacks to daily attacks
- Weakness may become permanent, especially after attacks in close succession

Diagnosis

Differential diagnosis
- Hyperkalemic periodic paralysis
- Myotonia congenita
- Paramyotonia congenita
- Myotonic dystrophy
- Schwartz-Jampel syndrome

History
- Symptoms last from hours up to several days
- Ocular, bulbar, and respiratory muscles are usually not affected
- Attacks occur with more frequency upon awakening and during/after vigorous exercise

Examination
- Not associated with clinical myotonia
- Lower limb weakness may be episodic or due to the slowly progressive permanent weakness that may develop

Testing
- Genetic testing
- Serum potassium levels do not correlate with the severity of weakness, and may be decreased or normal
- Serum creatine kinase levels rise during attacks
- EMG: compound muscle action potential (CMAP) amplitudes decrease during attack and increase after exercise; myotonic discharges typically absent
- Electrocardiogram: evidence of hypokalemia (flattened T-wave and ST-segment depression)

Pitfalls
- Aspiration pneumonia has caused death in several persons with HypoKPP

Red flags
- Avoid volatile anesthetic agents and depolarizing muscle relaxants in general anesthesia due to risk of postanesthesia weakness and malignant hyperthermia

Treatment

Medical
- Genetic counseling
- Diet rich in potassium and low in sodium and carbohydrates
- Oral (or IV) potassium supplementation

Exercise
- Gentle exercise

Modalities
- None indicated

Surgical
- None indicated

Consults
- Neurology

Complications of treatment
- Side effects of medications

Prognosis
- Lifespan is generally not affected

Helpful Hint
- Patients with diabetes should avoid acetazolamide, as it increases potassium uptake into muscle cells

Suggested Reading
Finsterer J. Primary periodic paralyses. *Acta Neurol Scand.* 2008;117:145–158.

Limb-Girdle Muscular Dystrophies

Nathan D. Prahlow MD

Description

The limb-girdle muscular dystrophies (LGMD) are a class of muscular dystrophies which predominantly affect the muscles of the shoulder and hip regions.

Etiology/Types

- Autosomal dominant
- Autosomal recessive
- Can be a new mutation

Epidemiology

- Rare
- LGMD2A is the most common type

Pathogenesis

- Over 20 chromosomal abnormalities are currently recognized, affecting many different muscle proteins

Risk Factors

- Family history positive for a limb-girdle muscular dystrophy

Clinical Features

- Proximal limb muscle weakness
- Dysarthria
- Modestly elevated serum creatine kinase (CK) levels, although some may show extreme elevation

Natural History

- Gradual progression of weakness over time
- Onset most common between age 8 and 15 years

Diagnosis

Differential diagnosis

- Duchenne muscular dystrophy
- Becker muscular dystrophy
- Fascioscapulohumeral dystrophy
- Congenital myopathies
- Polymyositis
- Autoimmune rippling muscle disease

History

- Any age of onset, but most common between age groups 8 and 15 years

- Cardiomyopathy
- Respiratory status
- Vision changes

Examination

- Proximal upper limb girdle weakness, including scapular winging
- Proximal posterior lower limb (hamstring/buttock) weakness
- Waddling gait
- Prominent contractures of Achilles, elbows, and spine
- Percussion-induced repetitive contractures—"rippling muscles"
- May develop cataracts

Testing

- Serum creatine kinase
- Muscle biopsy with histology and immunoanalysis
- Genetic testing
- Forced vital capacity—preserved in the most common type (LGMD2A)

Pitfalls

- Misdiagnosis of polmyositis due to increased CK and inflammatory infiltrate on muscle biopsy
- Missing cardiac involvement

Red flags

- Cardiac arrhythmias, cardiomyopathy, and respiratory failure risk, especially in types LGMD1B, LGMD2C-2F, and LGMD2I

Treatment

Medical treatment

- Supportive
- Assistive devices
- Genetic counseling
- Family tree surveillance

Exercise

- Stretching
- Prevention of contractures

Modalities
- Supportive

Surgical
- Automatic implanted cardiac defibrillator placement
- Cataract removal

Consults
- Cardiology
- Ophthalmology
- Neurology
- Physical medicine and rehabilitation

Complications of treatment
- Complications of surgery

Prognosis
- Patients with LGMD2A have normal lifespan

Helpful Hint
- Although CK levels may be high, this disease is not responsive to steroids

Suggested Reading
Bushby K. Diagnosis and management of the limb girdle muscular dystrophies. *Practical Neurol.* 2009;(9):314–323.

McArdle's Disease (Glycogen Storage Disease Type V)

Matthew Axtman DO

Description

McArdle's disease is a metabolic disorder caused by the inability to break down glycogen into glucose, resulting in exercise intolerance.

Etiology/Types

- Autosomal recessive
- Types:
  - Classic
  - Late-onset (rare)
  - Fatal infantile (rare)

Epidemiology

- Frequency is 1 per 100,000 births
- May be underdiagnosed due to mild symptoms in some patients

Pathogenesis

- Caused by the enzyme deficiency of myophosphorylase
- During exercise, glycogen is broken down into glucose via the myophosphorylase enzyme for the production of adenosine triphosphate (ATP)
- In McArdle's disease, initial energy is maintained by glucose in the blood, but once the blood-borne stores are depleted, there is an inability to convert the glycogen to glucose for utilization.

Risk Factors

- A positive family history of McArdle's disease

Clinical Features

- Patients note the inability to perform activities at normal levels
- Disease severity can range from mild exercise intolerance to fixed muscle weakness with severely limited activities of daily living
- Patients may display a "second wind" phenomenon in which they are able to resume activities at normal levels after a brief period of rest. This is due to the body's ability to use other sources of energy, such as fatty acids.

Natural History

- Symptoms usually present in the 2nd to 3rd decade of life

Diagnosis

Differential diagnosis

- Tarui disease (glycogen storage disease type VII)
- Glucose intolerance
- Glucose-6-phosphatase deficiency
- Glucose-6-phosphate dehydrogenase deficiency
- Hypoglycemia

History

- Exercise intolerance
- Myalgia
- Muscle cramps
- Fatigue
- Dark urine

Examination

- Muscle atrophy
- Proximal muscle weakness after exercise

Testing

- Elevated creatine kinase
- Urinalysis demonstrates myoglobinuria
- Muscle biopsy shows excess glycogen and absence of myophosphorylase
- Ischemic and nonischemic forearm exercise test: Hand is exercised for 30 seconds, with baseline and serial laboratory studies drawn, measuring lactate and ammonia levels

Pitfalls

- Delayed diagnosis that may cause rhabdomyolysis and renal failure if the patient continues to exercise at a high level

Red flags

- Rhabdomyolysis
- Renal failure

Treatment

Medical

- High carbohydrate diet may improve exercise tolerance
- Recommend having glucose supplementation for energy replacement
- Vitamin B6 supplementation

Exercises

- Patients are recommended to participate in moderate aerobic activity to improve exercise tolerance
- Avoid strenuous isometric or sustained aerobic exercises, which may lead to rhabdomyolysis

Modalities

- None

Surgical

- None

Consults

- Physical medicine and rehabilitation
- Nephrology
- Internal medicine

Complications of treatment

- None

Prognosis

- Benign process if strenuous activity is avoided
- May develop acute renal failure if excessive exercise is performed
- Older patients may develop fixed proximal muscle weakness

Helpful Hints

- The primary goal is activity and exercise modification
- Educate the patient on "second wind" phenomenon

Suggested Readings

Lucia A, Nogales-Gadea G, Perez M, et al. McArdle disease: What do neurologists need to know? *Nat Clin Pract Neurol.* 2008;4(10):568–577.

Quinlivan R, Buckley J, James M, Twist A, et al. McArdle disease: A clinical review. *J Neurol Neurosurg Psychiatry.* 2010;81(11):1182–1188. [Epub 2010 Sep 22].

Myotonia Congenita

Nathan D. Prahlow MD

Description

An inherited condition characterized by myotonia—the slow relaxation of a muscle after a contraction

Etiology/Types

- Thomsen's myotonia congenita: autosomal dominant inheritance
- Becker's myotonia congenita: autosomal recessive inheritance

Epidemiology

- 1 in 100,000 people

Pathogenesis

- Mutation in the CLCN1 gene, which encodes a protein found in the skeletal muscle chloride ion channels

Risk Factors

- Family history of myotonia congenita

Clinical Features

- Myotonia
- Stiffness, especially when first starting an activity
- After warm-up, muscles function may be normal
- "Little Hercules" presentation, with significant muscle hypertrophy at a young age

Natural History

- Early childhood presentation, with parent noting weakness, clumsiness, and/or stiffness in child (Becker's myotonia congenita appears at a later age than Thomsen's myotonia congenita)
- Symptoms may improve with age, but usually do not resolve

Diagnosis

Differential diagnosis

- Myotonic dystrophy
- Schwartz-Jampel syndrome
- Hyperkalemic periodic paralysis
- Paramyotonia congenita

History

- Developmentally "clumsy"
- Childhood gagging and difficulty swallowing
- Warm-up effect
- Becker's myotonia congenita: muscle stiffness and pain; temporary attacks of weakness

Examination

- Clinical myotonia
- Delayed release of handshake
- Forceful eye closing: delay in opening initially, but improves with repetition
- Becker's myotonia congenita: mild permanent weakness
- May have increased muscle bulk

Testing

- Genetic testing
- EMG: electrical myotonia; decrement with repetitive stimulation

Pitfalls

- Patients appear normal, but may have difficulties with some tasks and activities

Red flags

- None

Treatment

Medical

- Sodium channel blocker, such as mexiletine or phenytoin
- Medication use can be limited to times when the need for quicker action is predicted

Exercise

- Warm-up before a strenuous activity
- Therapy to address any activity of daily living or range-of-motion issues

Modalities

- As needed

Injection

- None indicated

Surgical
- None indicated

Consults
- Physical medicine and rehabilitation
- Neurology

Complications of treatment
- Side effects of medication

Prognosis
- Normal longevity

Helpful Hints
- Classic myotonia symptoms improve with physical activity
- Both clinical and electrical myotonia are seen in this disease process

Suggested Readings
Kurihara T. New classification and treatment for myotonic disorders. *Intern Med*, 2005:44(10):1027–1032.

Miller TM. Differential diagnosis of myotonic disorders. *Muscle Nerve* 2008;37:293–299.

VI: Muscle Diseases

Myotonic Dystrophy

Matthew Axtman DO

Description

Myotonic dystrophy [dystrophia myotonica (DM)] is a slowly progressive, variable disease characterized by muscle weakness, muscle atrophy, and myotonia. The disease also involves disorders of the cardiac, respiratory, ocular, neurologic, digestive, and endocrine systems.

Etiology/Types

- Autosomal dominant
- Types:
  - DM Type 1—Steinert's disease
  - DM Type 2—Proximal myotonic myopathy

Epidemiology

- Type 1—1 in 8,000 individuals
- Type 2—unknown

Pathogenesis

- Myotonic dystrophy type 1:
  - A trinucleotide (CTG) repeat disorder on chromosome 19
  - Mutation in the DMPK gene
  - 50 to 4000 repeats of the trinucleotide (healthy individuals have 5–37 repeats)
- Myotonic dystrophy type 2:
  - A tetranucleotide (CCTG) repeat disorder on chromosome 3
  - Mutation in the ZNF9 gene
  - 75 to 11,000 repeats of the tetranucleotide (healthy individuals have fewer than 75 repeats)

Risk Factors

- Family history of myotonic dystrophy

Clinical Features

- Progressive weakness in distal muscles in DM1 and in proximal muscles in DM2
- Myotonia-delayed relaxation of skeletal muscles after voluntary contraction
- Muscle atrophy
- Weight loss
- Swallowing difficulties
- Breathing difficulties
- Cardiac arrhythmias
- Abnormal facies—"Hatchet face," with tented open mouth and elongated face
- Vision changes
- Learning disabilities

Natural History

- There is a significantly high rate of variability with regard to age at symptom onset, severity of symptoms, and systems affected
- The disease is slowly progressive over years

Diagnosis

Differential diagnosis

- Paramyotonia congenita
- Congenital myotonia
- Limb-girdle dystrophy
- Polymositis
- Dermatomyositis
- Mild tetanus

History

- Progressive weakening of facial, jaw, neck, hand, and distal leg muscles in DM1
- Progressive weakening of neck, shoulder, hip flexor, and upper leg muscles in DM2
- Muscle pain
- Difficulty relaxing grip after grabbing or holding an object
- Hypersomnia
- Coughing/choking while eating or drinking
- Heart palpitations
- Developmental delays
- Weight loss
- Diarrhea
- Constipation
- Behavioral difficulties
- Infertility
- Early menopause

Examination

- Muscle weakness in the facial, neck, hand, distal leg muscles in DM1
- Muscle weakness in the neck, shoulder, hip flexor, and proximal leg muscles in DM2
- Muscle atrophy
- Myotonia
- Long face
- Bland facial expression

- Temple balding
- Stiff gait
- Dental malocclusion
- Poor suck reflex
- Ptosis
- Cardiac arrhythmias—atrial fibrillation/flutter most common
- Weak cough
- Muscle pain
- Gonadal atrophy
- Dental caries
- Pilomatrixoma tumors

Testing
- DNA testing
- Creatine kinase
- Electrocardiogram
- Holter monitor
- Echocardiogram
- Fasting blood glucose
- HgbA1c
- Testosterone, luteinizing hormone, follicle stimulating hormone levels
- Chest x-ray
- Pulmonary function testing
- Swallow assessment
- Muscle biopsy
- EMG
- Neuropsychological testing
- Sleep study
- Neuroimaging
- Invasive electrophysiologic testing

Pitfalls
- Patients may develop aspiration pneumonia if difficulty with swallowing is present
- Sudden cardiac death may occur in asymptomatic children

Red flags
- Cardiac and respiratory problems are the main causes of mortality
- Increased risk of mortality with anesthesia
- Increased sensitivity to drugs that decrease respiratory drive

Treatment

Medical
- Evaluation for orthoses, assistive devices, and adaptive equipment
- Non-steroidal anti-inflammatory drugs for pain

- Cough assist devices
- Pacemaker/implantable cardioverter defibrillator
- Continuous positive airway pressure
- Hormone replacement therapy
- Antidiabetic drugs
- Dietary management
- Incentive spirometry
- Mexiletine for disabling myotonia

Exercises
- Range of motion
- Strengthening
- Aerobic exercise
- Aquatic therapy

Modalities
- Heat for muscle pain
- Patients may need heated gloves during cold weather to help prevent myotonia

Surgical
- Cataract extraction
- Blepharoplasty
- Pilomatrixoma removal

Consults
- Cardiology
- Pulmonology
- Endocrinology
- Physical medicine and rehabilitation
- Neurology
- Ophthalmology
- Gastroenterology
- Neuropsychology

Complications of treatment
- Vigorous activity should be avoided due to the risk of sudden cardiac death
- Antiarrhythmics and antimyotonic medication should be prescribed carefully due to proarrhythmic effects

Prognosis
- Disability is more severe, the earlier the symptoms appear in life
- Increased length of the repeat disorder is associated with worse prognosis and earlier life expectancy
- Severity of the disease increases and prognosis worsens with successive generations

Helpful Hints
- Patients may have very mild symptoms and go undiagnosed until a child is born and is diagnosed with the disorder

- The symptoms are highly variable depending on the number of associated repeats on the chromosome
- Myotonic dystrophy is associated with insulin resistance leading to diabetes mellitus

Suggested Readings

Kurihara T. New classification and treatment for myotonic disorders. *Intern Med.* 2005;44:1027–1032.

Orngreen MC, Olsen DB, Vissing J. Aerobic training in patients with myotonic dystrophy type 1. *Ann. Neurol.* 2005;57:754–757.

Turner C, Hilton-Jones D. The myotonic dystrophies: diagnosis and management. *J Neurol Neurosurg Psychiatry.* 2010;81(4):358–367.

Paramyotonia Congenita

Nathan D. Prahlow MD

Description
Also known as Eulenberg syndrome. Characterized by paradoxical myotonia, in which the myotonic activity is heightened by activity

Etiology/Types
- Autosomal dominant

Epidemiology
- 1 in 200,000 or rarer; locally may be more common due to founder effect

Pathogenesis
- Mutation in the α-subunit of the muscular sodium channel gene SCN4A

Risk Factors
- Positive family history

Clinical Features
- Cold-induced localized prolonged myotonia and weakness
- Increased myotonia with repetitive or continual activity
- Facial muscles and upper limb muscles more involved

Natural History
- Onset in childhood
- Nonprogressive
- Weakness from paramyotonia congenita is not permanent

Diagnosis

Differential diagnosis
- Hyperkalemic periodic paralysis
- Myotonia congenita
- Myotonic dystrophy
- Schwartz-Jampel syndrome

History
- Symptoms after cold exposure
- Symptoms after vigorous exercise
- Flaccid weakness may follow the episodes of myotonia
- Symptoms may last minutes to several hours

Examination
- Paradoxical myotonia: rapidly repeated forcible eye closure brings on the inability to open eyes
- No muscular wasting or hypertrophy

Testing
- Genetic testing
- Serum potassium moderately elevated; serum creatine kinase (CK) usually elevated
- EMG: plentiful myotonic discharges present during cooling of the muscle

Pitfalls
- Misdiagnosis

Red flags
- None

Treatment

Medical treatment
- Mexiletine, a sodium channel blocker, may be taken during cold-weather months
- Chlorothiazide and acetazolamide have been shown to be helpful

Exercise
- Strenuous exercise may trigger or worsen symptoms

Modalities
- None indicated

Injection
- None indicated

Surgical
- None indicated

Consults
- Neurology

Complications of treatment
- Side effects of medication

Prognosis
- No impact on lifespan

Helpful Hint
- Cold triggers also include swimming in cold water, cold drafts, and eating ice cream

Suggested Readings
Kurihara T. New classification and treatment for myotonic disorders. *Intern Med.* 2005;44(10):1027–1032.
Miller TM. Differential diagnosis of myotonic disorders. *Muscle Nerve.* 2008;37:293–299.

Polymyositis

Gabriel Smith MD ■ Nathan D. Prahlow MD

Description
An inflammatory myopathy characterized by symmetric proximal weakness

Etiology/Types
■ Unknown

Epidemiology
■ Approximately 1 in 250,000
■ Female-to-male ratio of 2:1
■ Affects adults > 18 years old
■ Extremely rare in children

Pathogenesis
■ Thought to be initiated by viral illness or an autoimmune response, resulting in muscle destruction

Risk Factors
■ Age 40 to 60 years
■ Female
■ Presence of connective tissue diseases

Clinical Features
■ Gradual muscle weakness and myalgias
■ Systemic symptoms: fever, malaise, arthralgias
■ Dysphagia and/or dysphonia
■ Pulmonary dysfunction

Natural History
■ Unknown agent causes insult to muscles leading to release of autoantigens
■ Antigens are presented to CD8+ T cells
■ Activated CD8+ T cells directly damage muscles through release of cytokines
■ Macrophages also contribute to inflammation
■ Sufficient damage leads to muscle destruction and weakness over several months

Diagnosis
Differential diagnosis
■ Dermatomyositis
■ Inclusion body myositis
■ Polymyalgia rheumatica
■ Hypothyroidism
■ Systemic lupus erythematosis
■ Fibromyalgia

History
■ Symmetric proximal muscle weakness, increasing over 3 to 6 months
■ Many patients have prior history of connective tissue diseases
■ Myalgias
■ Fatigue, fever, anorexia
■ May have respiratory or gastrointestinal complaints depending on what muscle groups are involved

Examination
■ Symmetric weakness, proximal > distal
■ Tenderness of involved muscles
■ Deep tendon reflexes and sensation preserved

Testing
■ Erythrocyte sedimentation rate (ESR)
■ Complete blood count (CBC)
■ Anti-nuclear antibody (ANA)
■ Anti Jo-1 antibodies
■ Serum creatine kinase
■ EMG
■ Chest x-ray
■ Muscle biopsy

Pitfalls
■ Due to insidious onset, symptoms may be disregarded as mere fatigue, delaying treatment

Red flags
■ Respiratory distress/failure
■ Dysphagia and dysphonia
■ Aspiration pneumonia

Treatment
Medical
The typical sequence of treatment is:
■ High-dose prednisone
■ Azithropine or methotrexate for steroid sparing
■ Intravenous immunoglobulin (IVIg)
■ Rituximab, cyclosporine, cyclophosphamide, or tacrolimus

Exercises

- Physical therapy—passive range of motion and splinting help prevent contraction
- Aerobic exercise during inactive phase
- Speech therapy to prevent aspiration

Modalities

- Heat for muscle pain

Surgical

- None.

Consults

- Neurology
- Rheumatology
- Cardiology
- Pulmonology
- Physical medicine and rehabilitation
- Physical therapy/occupational therapy (PT/OT), speech therapy

Complications of treatment

- Steroids, immunosuppressants, and chemotherapeutic agents are notorious for their side-effect profiles

Prognosis

- Five-year survival is 95%, 10-year survival is 84%
- Worse prognosis with advanced age, female, presence of Anti-Jo-1 and Anti-SRP antibodies
- Also worse prognosis if associated with cardiac or pulmonary dysfunction

Helpful Hints

- Most patients improve with therapy
- Many make full functional recovery
- Patients with associated interstitial lung disease greatly benefit from cyclophosphamide

Suggested Readings

Dalakas MC. Polymyositis, dermatomyositis, and inclusion body myositis. *Harrison's Principles of Internal Medicine.* 17th ed. New York: McGraw Hill; 2008.

Dalakas MC. Inflammatory muscle diseases: A critical review on pathogenesis and therapies. *Curr Opin Pharmacol.* 2010;10(3):346–352.

Pompe Disease (Glycogen Storage Disease Type II)

Matthew Axtman DO

Description
Pompe disease is a metabolic disorder caused by the accumulation of glycogen within lysosomes causing progressive muscle weakness.

Etiology/Types
- Autosomal recessive
- Types:
  - Infantile (4–8 months old)
  - Late onset (>1 year old)

Epidemiology
- Frequency is 1 per 138,000 births for infantile type
- Frequency is 1 per 57,000 for late onset type

Pathogenesis
- Caused by a deficiency of the lysosomal enzyme acid alpha-glucosidase (also called acid maltase)

Risk Factors
- A positive family history of Pompe disease

Clinical Features
- Patients with the infantile form present with weakness, hypotonia, respiratory infections, delayed milestones, feeding difficulties, and failure to thrive
- Patients with the late-onset form present with progressive muscle weakness, recurrent respiratory infections, difficulty swallowing, and delayed milestones
- Young children may not be able to walk, run, and jump at the same age as their peers

Natural History
- The infantile form progresses quickly and patients have a high mortality if left untreated
- There is a glycogen buildup within cardiac muscles that causes cardiac hypertrophy in the infantile type
- There is a progressive weakness of respiratory muscles that leads to an ineffective cough, difficulty in breathing, recurrent respiratory infections, and respiratory failure
- The late-onset-type progresses slowly and is highly variable
- Patients with the late-onset type may have a mild disability for years or develop the need for assistive devices for mobility and ventilation

Diagnosis

Differential diagnosis
- Duchenne muscular dystrophy
- Spinal muscular atrophy
- Limb-girdle dystrophy
- Inflammatory myopathies
- Amyotrophic lateral sclerosis

History
- Infants have difficulty lifting head or rolling over
- Failure to gain weight
- Delayed or failure to meet developmental milestones
- Progressive decrease in limb strength
- Recurrent respiratory infections
- Difficulty chewing and swallowing
- Frequent falls
- Difficulty climbing stairs or standing
- Difficulty breathing, especially while lying down

Examination
- Hypotonia
- Head lag
- Weak suck reflex
- Weakness of leg and pelvic muscles
- Hepatomegaly
- Enlarged tongue
- Waddling gait
- Loss of balance with ambulation
- Scoliosis
- Abnormal heart rhythm

Testing
- Acid alpha-glucosidase enzyme levels
- Creatine kinase levels are elevated
- Muscle biopsy—excessive glycogen accumulation
- Chest x-ray—heart is enlarged
- Electrocardiogram

- Echocardiogram—thickened cardiac tissue
- EMG
- Pulmonary function tests—decreased vital capacity
- Sleep study

Pitfalls
- Failure to monitor respiratory status
- Failure to monitor nutritional status

Red flags
- Recurrent respiratory infections
- Failure to gain weight
- Loss of vital capacity

Treatment

Medical
- Enzyme replacement therapy using Alglucosidase alfa
  - Myozyme is approved for infantile-type Pompe disease
  - Lumizyme is approved for late-onset type Pompe disease for patients 8 years and older who do not have evidence of cardiac hypertrophy
- Evaluation for bracing, orthotics, and assistive devices
- Ventilatory support

Exercises
- Strengthening of weakened limb muscles
- Strengthening of respiratory and oropharyngeal muscles
- Range of motion and stretching to prevent contracture formation
- Developing motor skills

Modalities
- None

Surgical
- Spinal fusion for severe scoliosis
- Tendon release for contractures

Consults
- Cardiology
- Neurology
- Pulmonology
- Respiratory therapy
- Speech therapy
- Genetic counseling
- Orthopedics

Complications of treatment
- Physical therapy should not exceed exercise tolerance and compromise the patient's cardiac or respiratory status

Prognosis
- Variable, depending on the type, age of onset, and severity of symptoms
- Infantile type is usually fatal within the first 2 years of life due to cardiorespiratory failure
- Without medical treatment, the disease is lethal in infants and young children
- Late-onset type is slowly progressive and associated with significant morbidity and premature mortality
- Prognosis is dependent on respiratory status

Helpful Hints
- Respiratory status should be monitored every 3 to 6 months for decline of function
- Pompe disease is the only glycogen storage disease with a defect in lysosomal metabolism
- Cardiac involvement in the late-onset type is lacking or mild compared with the infantile form

Suggested Readings
Hirschhorn R, Reuser AJJ. Glycogen storage disease type II: Acid alpha-glucosidase (acid maltase) deficiency. In: Scriver C, Beaudet A, Sly W, Valle D, eds. *The Metabolic and Molecular Bases of Inherited Disease.* 8th ed. (pp. 3389–3420). New York: McGraw-Hill; 2001.

Wang RY, Bodamer OA, Watson MS, Wilcox WR; on behalf of the ACMG Work Group on Diagnostic Confirmation of Lysosomal Storage Diseases. Lysosomal storage diseases: Diagnostic confirmation and management of presymptomatic individuals. *Genet Med.* 2011;13(5):457–484.

VI: Muscle Diseases

Rhabdomyolysis

Gabriel Smith MD ■ Nathan D. Prahlow MD

Description
Breakdown of striated muscle fibers with the release of potentially toxic cellular contents into the systemic circulation

Etiology/Types
- There are many causes of rhabdomyolysis
- Major categories include drugs/toxins, trauma, exertion, immobilization, muscle hypoxia, genetic defects, infections, and extreme body temperature changes
- HMG-CoA reductase inhibitors—"Statins"
  - This class of medication has widespread use
  - Generally very safe and well tolerated
  - Subclinical muscle pain and weakness may affect 7% of patients on statin monotherapy
  - Clinically detectable myopathy incidence of less than 0.1%, and only one fatal rhabdomyolysis case per 5 million patients taking statins

Epidemiology
- Accounts for 7% to 10% of acute kidney injury (AKI)
- Overall more common in adults
- Somewhat higher prevalence in males

Pathogenesis
- Muscle cell death releases toxic cell components, resulting in end organ damage

Risk Factors
- See "Etiology" section

Clinical Features
- Highly variable, subclinical to severe
- Weakness, myalgias
- Dark urine
- Altered mental status if severe

Natural History
- Some insult results in muscle cell death
- Electrolyte disturbances result from release of intracellular contents
- Damaged muscle cells retain water, resulting in hypovolemia
- Hypovolemia activates the sympathetic nervous system and other systems resulting in renal vasoconstriction and renal ischemia
- Myoglobin released from muscle cells is toxic to renal tubules, resulting in AKI

Diagnosis

Differential diagnosis
- Acute intermittent porphyria
- Sickle cell crisis
- Viral myopathy
- Compartment syndrome
- Diabetic ketoacidosis

History
- History depends on etiology
- Many patients notice dark urine
- Myalgias and weakness
- Flu like symptoms
- Oliguria

Examination
- Ranges from benign to serious
- Muscle tenderness or rigidity
- Fever or low body temperature
- Signs of sepsis

Testing
- Serum creatine kinase repeated every 6 to 12 hrs until peak is measured
- Urine dipstick for blood
- Fractional excretion of sodium
- Basic metabolic panel
- Cardiac troponins
- Complete blood count
- Coagulation studies
- Electrocardiogram

Pitfalls
- May have insidious onset, especially in immobile hospitalized patients with other comorbidities

Red flags
- Cardiac arrhythmias
- Signs of compartment syndrome
- Signs of disseminated intravascular coagulation

Treatment

Medical
- Treat underlying condition
- Vigorous hydration with isotonic crystalloids
- Loop diuretics
- Mannitol may reduce compartment pressures
- Consider bicarbonate if serious acidosis exists
- Treat electrolyte imbalances appropriately

Exercises
- Avoid extreme exercise as this can precipitate rhabdomyolysis

Modalities
- Heat may relieve residual myalgias

Injection
- None

Surgical
- Necessary in case of compartment syndrome

Consults
- Nephrology:
  - Hematology
  - Internal Medicine

Complications of treatment
- Aggressive hydration may result in fluid overload, leading to respiratory complaints

Prognosis
- Prognosis depends on underlying etiology and any other existing comorbidities
- Significantly worse if renal failure results

Helpful Hints
- Early intervention is important for preventing renal failure
- Focus treatment on underlying cause of rhabdomyolysis
- Always consider rhabdomyolysis as possible cause of renal failure in chronic illness patients

Suggested Reading
Bosch X, Poch E, Grau JM: Rhabdomyolysis and acute kidney injury. *New Engl J Med.* 2009;361:62–72.

VI: Muscle Diseases

Schwartz-Jampel Syndrome

Nathan D. Prahlow MD

Description

Also known as dysostosis enchondralis metaepiphysaria, chondrodystrophic myotonia, and osteochondromuscular dystrophy, the Schwartz-Jampel syndrome (SJS) includes features of muscle stiffness and mild weakness, characteristic facies, and bony deformities

Etiology/Types

- Type IA: most common
- Type IB: apparent at birth
- Type II: a separate disorder, known as Stuve-Wiedemann syndrome

Epidemiology

- Unknown

Pathogenesis

- Mutations of the HSPG2 gene, causing abnormalities in the basement membrane protein perlecan

Risk Factors

- Family history of SJS

Clinical Features

- Muscle stiffness and mild weakness
- Characteristic facies: small, fixed facial features
- Bony deformities: short stature, joint contractures
- Intelligence may be affected, but high intelligence may be seen

Natural History

- Usually diagnosed before 3 years of age
- Motor developmental delay, particularly ambulation
- Gait becomes progressively stiff and wide based
- Slowly progressive, but may be static

Diagnosis

Differential diagnosis

- Myotonia congenita
- Myotonic dystrophy
- Muscular dystrophies
- Hereditary motor-sensory neuropathies
- Myasthenia gravis
- Periodic paralysis
- Stiff man syndrome

History

- Neonates/infants: feeding difficulty, choking, respiratory failure
- Motor developmental delay, especially ambulation

Examination

- Facies: small palpebral fissures (blepharophimosis), low-set ears, small puckered mouth, micrognathia, and hypertrichosis of the eyelids (excess hair, or multiple rows of eyelashes)
- Short neck, pigeon breast, protuberant abdomen
- Sparse subcutaneous tissue
- Clinical myotonia with action and percussion
- Joint contractures of shoulders, elbows, wrists
- Muscle mass may be atrophic or hypertrophic

Testing

- Genetic studies
- EMG: usually normal nerve conduction study (NCS); spontaneous high-frequency/low-voltage discharges at rest, which increase with needle movement, muscle percussion, or voluntary movement; may resemble myotonic discharges
- Mild to moderate creatine kinase elevation
- Muscle biopsy: normal or nonspecific myopathic abnormalities
- Plain films to document bony abnormalities noted on examination
- Occasional electrocardiogram abnormalities

Pitfalls

- Mistaken diagnosis

Red flags

- Type II (Stuve-Wiedemann syndrome) has a high-infant mortality rate

Treatment

Medical treatment

- Anticonvulsants and quinine
- Antiarrhythmics

Exercise

- Maintenance of range of motion
- Massage
- Gradual muscle warm-up

Modalities
■ As needed

Injection
■ Botulinum toxin for those unable to maintain an open eye

Surgical
■ Orbicularis oculi myectomy, levator aponeurosis resection, and lateral canthopexy for severe blepharophimosis not amenable to botulinum toxin
■ Contracture release

Consults
■ Ophthalmology
■ Orthopedic surgery

Complications of treatment
■ Side effects of medications

Prognosis
■ Type IA does not significantly shorten lifespan
■ 20% of patients are mentally retarded

Helpful Hint
■ Although 20% are mentally retarded, many patients are of normal or superior intelligence

Suggested Readings
Ault J. Schwartz-Jampel syndrome treatment and management. (Updated February 2, 2010). http://emedicine.medscape.com/article/1172013-treatment#a1128. Medscape, New York.
Pascuzzi RM. Schwartz-Jampel syndrome. *Semin Neurol.* 1991;11(3):267–273.

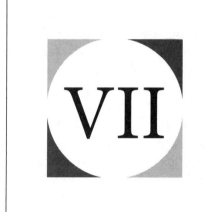

Movement Disorders

Blepharospasm

Susan X. Yu DO ▪ Nathan D. Prahlow MD

Description
A focal dystonia characterized by excessive involuntary repetitive blinking or sustained eyelid closure

Etiology/Types
- Also called benign essential blepharospasm
- Unknown etiology
- Autosomal dominant disorder with reduced penetrance of about 5% with genetic heterogeneity
- Due to spasms of orbicularis oculi (OO)
- Sometimes due to failure of levator palpebrae contraction: apraxia of eyelid opening

Epidemiology
- Average onset age 50 to 60 years
- 12 to 133 per million
- 2.3 times more frequent in women and with older onset age

Pathogenesis
- Unknown. Likely due to pathology in the basal ganglia, brainstem, and thalamus
- Dry eye and photophobia suggest trigeminal system sensitization and/or sympathetically maintained pain

Risk Factors
- Increased risk:
  - prior head trauma with loss of consciousness
  - family history of dystonia
  - prior eye disease
- Reduced risk:
  - previous cigarette smoking
  - coffee drinking

Clinical Features
- Begins gradually with excessive blinking and eye irritation (normal blink = once every 2 to 3 seconds)
- Eyelid spasms may occur with cervical dystonia, Meige syndrome, and other cranial dystonias (clenching or mouth opening, grimacing, and tongue protrusion)
- Triggers: dry eyes on bright light exposure, watching television, reading, driving, fatigue, and emotional stress
- Improved by concentrating on a specific task or by using sensory tricks (talking or touching the forehead or the eyebrow)

Natural History
- With progression, spasms occur frequently during the day, disappear in sleep, then reappear several hours after waking
- Further progression: spasms intensify to the degree that the patient is functionally blind, as the eyelids may remain forcibly closed for hours

Diagnosis

Differential diagnosis
- *Blepharitis*: eyelid inflammation
- Blepharoptosis: drooping of the eyelid margin
- Facial palsy: inability to close the upper lid and laxity of the lower lid
- Third nerve palsy
- Stroke
- Dry eye syndrome
- Orbital inflammatory syndrome
- Thyroid eye disease (due to overactive thyroid gland)
- Autoimmune diseases such as myasthenia gravis and multiple sclerosis

History
- Clinical diagnosis

Examination
- Observation of delayed eye opening

Testing
- EMG recordings of the pretarsal orbicularis oculi
- In eyelid apraxia, EMG shows levator muscle inactivity despite the patient's attempt to open eyes

Pitfalls
- Selective contraction of the pretarsal portion of the orbicularis oculi can be responsible for eyelid closure
- May be associated with a reactive depression

Red flags
- When accompanied by other symptoms of stroke, such as extremity weakness

Treatment

Medical
- Anticholinergics: trihexyphenidyl and benztropine
- Antihistamine: diphenhydramine
- Benzodiazepines: clonazepam, diazepam, lorazepam, alprazolam
- Antispasticity agents: baclofen and tizanidine
- Antipsychotics: haloperidol, thioridazine, amitriptyline
- New-generation neuroleptics: tetrabenazine, risperdone, olanzapine, quetiapine, and clozapine
- Others: Carbidopa/levodopa, carbamazepine, propranolol

Exercise
- Occupational therapy to work on stress reduction

Modalities
- Use of a sensory trick: glasses fitted with wire loops to press against the brow or to lift the upper lid (Lundie loops)
- Reduction of photophobia with FL-41 rose-tint lenses

Injection
- Treatment of choice: botulinum toxin injection of the eyelid muscles:
  - High efficacy for many years without side effect or loss of efficacy
  - Botox 27- to 30-gauge without EMG
  - Start with 1.25 to 2.5 units (0.1 mL)/muscle:
    - Upper lid: medial pretarsal OO
    - Upper Lid: lateral pretarsal OO
    - Lower lid: lateral pretarsal OO
  - Unless the pretarsal portion is injected with botulinum toxin, treatment will fail, and the patient could be diagnosed with apraxia in error. For proper diagnosis, inject Riolan's muscle, at the lid margin
- Doxorubicin chemomyectomy provides >10 years relief but has skin side effects
- Superior sympathetic ganglion blockade with local anesthetic to decrease photophobia

Surgical
- Myectomy of the eyelid protractors; shortening of the levator tendon or frontalis sling
- Deep brain stimulation for patients also with cranial dystonia—mild to 75% improvement

Consults
- Neurology
- Ophthalmology
- Neurosurgery

Complications of treatment
- Botulinum toxin: ptosis (21%), superficial punctate keratitis (6%), and eye dryness (6%)
- Anticholinergics and antihistamine: constipation, dry mouth, difficulty in urinating, trouble concentrating, memory loss, and confusion. Use caution with glaucoma
- Benzodiazepines and antispasticity agents: sleepiness, difficulty of thinking, fatigue, imbalance, dependency
- Antipsychotics: reversible parkinsonism, involuntary movements
- New-generation neuroleptics: sleepiness, insomnia, constipation, fatigue, and confusion; Clozaril can lower the white blood cell count

Prognosis
- Typically a chronic condition
- 10% spontaneously remit in the first 5 years
- More likely to spread past the head (31%) than upper extremity dystonias, most during the first 5 years

Helpful Hints
- Determine the contribution of lid opening apraxia because it does not respond well to botulinum toxin injections
- Add oral medications slowly when botulinum toxin injections are not effective, titrate to effective dosage to minimize side effects

Suggested Readings
Hallett M, Evinger C, Jankovic J, Stacy M, BEBRF International Workshop. Update on blepharospasm: Report from the BEBRF International Workshop. *Neurol.* 2008; 71(16):1275.
Hallett M. Blepharospasm: Recent advances. *Neurol.* 2002;59(9):1306–1312.

Dystonia

Shashank J. Davé DO FAAPMR

Description
Involuntary muscle contractions leading to abnormal movement and posture

Etiology/Types
- Primary dystonia: mostly inherited in autosomal dominant pattern
- Secondary dystonia: usually acquired and has an associated neurologic impairment and ataxia
- Focal: for example, cervical dystonia, blepharospasm, facial dystonia, occupational dystonia
- Generalized: involves one limb, trunk, and another body area
- Spasmodic dysphonia–laryngeal muscles

Epidemiology
- Wide range, based on few epidemiologic studies
- 2 to 7500 per million, with cervical dystonia being the most common focal dystonia

Pathogenesis
- Neurodegenerative disorder
- Type 1 (DYT1) dystonia: mutation in TOR1A gene which encodes an ATP-binding protein
- May involve basal ganglia, motor cortex, and cerebellum
- Decreased inhibition
- Neurotransmitter imbalance in dopamine and acetylcholine

Risk Factors
- Very few, but may be associated with stressful life-events

Clinical Features
- Muscle spasm with involuntary sustained tonic or clonic contractions
- Co-contraction: simultaneous agonist and antagonist contraction
- Contractions may intensify with voluntary effort
- Sensory trick: light touch over affected body region may attenuate dystonia

Natural History
- May begin in the head/neck or a limb, then progress to adjacent parts, such as the trunk
- Chronic, but some may spontaneously remiss

Diagnosis

Differential diagnosis
- Brain injury: acquired and congenital
- Stroke
- Multiple sclerosis
- Seizures
- Encephalitis
- Musculoskeletal disorders
- Drugs such as dopamine blockers
- Conversion disorder

History
- Abnormal contractions of the involved limb/body part during activity, which usually goes away with rest

Examination
- Depends on body part affected; *for head and neck, see Chapter 89 on "Torticollis"*
- Movement usually has a directional component
- Geste antagoniste: sensory trick such as light touch or brushing the involved area, which attenuates the movement

Testing
- Usually a clinical diagnosis
- Brain magnetic resonance imaging (MRI) to check for lesions in the basal ganglia, motor cortex, and cerebellum, and to rule out other diagnoses listed above
- Laboratories: comprehensive metabolic panel, complete blood count
- Wilson's disease: ceruloplasmin
- Gene testing for hereditary dystonia, such as DYT1 dystonia
- Levodopa trial: for dopa-responsive dystonia

Pitfalls
- Conversion disorder
- Essential tremor versus dystonia
- Dystonia plus parkinsonism

Red flags
- Neoplasm
- Cord compression: bilateral symptoms and lower limb involvement

Treatment

Medical
- Depends on etiology
- Levodopa, if trial is successful
- Trihexyphenidyl
- Baclofen: oral, intrathecal
- Clonazepam
- Tetrabenazine

Exercises
- Physical therapy for stretching and strengthening; gait retraining
- Occupational therapy for activities of daily living
- Generalized cardiovascular conditioning
- Contracture prevention

Modalities
- Ice/heat for pain
- Electrical stimulation for weakness

Injection
- Botulinum toxin for focal muscle overactivity
- Gene therapy: for DYT1 dystonia, which involves inhibiting gene expression; preclinical studies are promising

Surgical
- Neurosurgical for deep brain stimulation of internal globus pallidus or less commonly, subthalamic nucleus

Consults
- Movement disorder neurologist
- Genetic counselor (if appropriate)
- Physical medicine and rehabilitation

Complications of treatment
- Levodopa: dyskinesia, hypotension, hallucination
- Trihexyphenidyl: xerostomia, blurred vision, glaucoma
- Baclofen: sedation, dizziness; avoid sudden withdrawal
- Botulinum toxin: xerostomia, dysphagia, weakness

Prognosis
- Treatment largely symptomatic
- No curative treatments available
- Response rate to levodopa is 15%

Helpful Hint
- Generalized dystonia warrants generalized treatment, whereas focal dystonia warrants focal treatment

Suggested Readings
Comella CL, Pullman SL. Botulinum toxins in neurological disease. *Muscle Nerve.* 2004;29:628.
Geyer HL, Bressman SB. The diagnosis of dystonia. *Lancet Neurol.* 2006;5:780.
Janovic J. Treatment of dystonia. *Lancet Neurol.* 2006;5:864.
Simpson DM, Blitzer A, Brashear A, et al. Assessment: Botulinum neurotoxin for the treatment of movement disorders (an evidence-based review): Report of the Therapeutics and Technology Assessment Subcommittee of the American Academy of Neurology. *Neurol.* 2008;70:1699.

Essential Tremor

Susan X. Yu DO ■ Nathan D. Prahlow MD

Description

Progressive movement disorder, characterized by a rhythmic, involuntary, oscillatory shaking of body parts

Etiology/Types

- 50% are autosomal dominant

Epidemiology

- 0.4% to 6% prevalence; 5% of those over age 65 years
- Incidence increases with age
- Affects both genders, all ages, all ethnicities

Pathogenesis

- Unknown. Lewy bodies found in the brainstem (locus ceruleus) along with degenerative changes in the cerebellum

Risk Factors

- Each child of an affected parent has a 50% chance of inheritance
- No known environmental risk factor

Clinical Features

- An action tremor which is usually postural, but occasionally kinetic
- Action tremors occur during voluntary muscle contraction
  - Postural tremors occur while maintaining a position against gravity, such as when holding hands outstretched
  - Kinetic tremors (intention tremors) occur during target-directed movements
- Commonly affects wrists and hands, but also affects the head, lower extremities, and voice
- Either high or low tremor frequency, without other neurologic findings
- Relieved with alcohol (two drinks per day)

Natural History

- Any age of onset, often in early adulthood

Diagnosis

Differential diagnosis

- Essential tremor is a diagnosis of exclusion:
  - 4 to 8 Hz, low amplitude (less than 1 cm movement)

- Enhanced physiologic tremor:
  - Postural tremor, 10 to 12 Hz, low amplitude
  - Sudden onset
- Drug and metabolic-induced tremor:
  - Postural tremor, 10 to 12 Hz, low amplitude
  - Sudden onset
- Orthostatic tremor, 15 to 20 Hz
- Parkinsonism:
  - Resting tremor, 4 to 6 Hz, "pill-rolling"
  - Gradual onset in older patients
  - Micrographia
  - Gait: narrow-based and shuffling
- Cerebellar tremor/brain tumors:
  - Intention and postural tremor, low frequency
  - Ipsilateral to lesion
  - Abnormal finger-to-nose and heel-to-shin
  - Gait: wide-based and ataxic
- Psychogenic tremor:
  - Changing tremor frequency and amplitude
  - Abrupt onset, extinction with distraction
- Dystonic tremor:
  - Age younger than 50 years
  - Irregular, jerky tremors
  - Abnormal wrist flexion
- Wilson's disease:
  - Age younger than 40 years
  - "Wing-beating" tremor
- Fragile X syndrome

History

- Hand tremors noticeable by patient and family
- Handwriting change—view old handwriting samples to compare
- Precipitating and relieving factors, such as caffeine, alcohol, medications, exercise, fatigue, or stress

Examination

- Examine for tremors at rest and with activity:
  - Head: nod and shake head
  - Jaw, tongue
  - Voice: Reciting a standard paragraph and enunciating a sustained vowel
  - Limbs:
    - Outstretching arms with wrist supination and pronation

- Apposing index fingers one inch apart in front of the face
- Performing finger-to-nose, shin-to-heel
- Drinking or pouring from a paper cup
■ Handwriting samples: large, tremulous, angulated loops; Archimedes spirals
■ Normal gait, Romberg, and muscle tone

Testing

■ Laboratories: Rule out potential metabolic or toxin causes with thyroid stimulating hormone, serum ceruloplasmin, 24-hour urinary copper, complete blood count with differential, comprehensive metabolic profile
■ Imaging: Rule out other potential causes such as Parkinson's disease with brain computed tomography/magnetic resonance imaging (CT/MRI), single photon emission computed tomography (SPECT) to visualize the dopaminergic pathways

Pitfalls

■ Sleep disorders may cause fatigue, which amplifies physiologic tremors
■ Polyneuropathy may cause small involuntary movements that mimic tremors

Red flags

■ Seizures, fever, and anemia may indicate other causes of tremor

Treatment

Medical

■ Propranolol: 50% of patients benefit
■ Primidone: 50% of patients benefit
■ Topiramate: 50% of patients benefit
■ The above can sometimes be used in combination
■ Gabapentin

Exercises

■ None

Modalities

■ Weighted utensils may help dampen tremor for self-feeding

Injection

■ Botulinum toxin is effective for head tremors
■ Botulinum toxin has varying results for voice tremors

Surgical

■ Deep brain stimulation (DBS):
  – Nucleus ventrointermedius of the thalamus and neighboring subthalamic structures highly effective, but gradual loss of tremor control

■ Bilateral DBS more effective for voice tremors, but dysphagia and dysarthria are more likely as side effects
■ Thalamotomy:
  – Radiofrequency ablation
  – Gamma knife

Consults

■ Neurology
■ Neurosurgery

Complications of treatment

■ Medications:
  – Propranolol: bradycardia, syncope, fatigue, and erectile dysfunction
  – Primidone: drowsiness, dizziness, and disequilibrium
  – Topiramate: weight loss, extremity paresthesias, and memory disturbance
■ Deep brain stimulation:
  – Dysarthria 3% to 18%, paresthesias 6% to 36%, dystonia 2% to 9%, balance disturbance 3% to 8%, ataxia 6%, and limb weakness 4% to 8%
■ Hardware complications 25%

Prognosis

■ Progressive disorder
■ Tremor amplitude increases with age
■ Tremor frequency decreases with age
■ 25% of patients retire early or modify their career path

Helpful Hints

■ Tremor are categorized by activating condition (kinetic/intention, postural, resting, and isometric), topographical distribution (head, voice, and limbs), and frequency (low <4 Hz, medium 4 to 7 Hz, and high >7 Hz)
■ Many medications can influence or cause tremors by increasing adrenergic activity
■ Physiological states, such as anxiety, excitement, fright, muscle fatigue, thyrotoxicosis, fever, and pheochromocytoma, may influence tremor severity

Suggested Readings

Crawford P, Zimmerman EE. Differentiation and diagnosis of tremor. *Am Fam Physician.* 2011;83(6):697–702. (Review).

Deuschl G, Raethjen J, Hellriegel H, Elble R. Treatment of patients with essential tremor. *Lancet Neurol.* 2011;10(2): 148–161. (Review).

VII: Movement Disorders

Friedreich's Ataxia (Primary Spinocerebellar Degeneration)

Susan X. Yu DO ■ Shashank J. Davé DO FAAPMR

Description

An inherited disease that causes progressive degeneration of the nervous system resulting in ataxia, muscle weakness, areflexia, and heart disease

Etiology/Types

- Hereditary: autosomal recessive
- Defect in chromosome 9 with hyperexpansion of GAA repeats in intron 1 of frataxin gene

Epidemiology

- Ratio of 1:50,000 white
- Ratio of 1:60 to 1:100 carrier frequency

Pathogenesis

- Mitochondrial protein frataxin is severely reduced due to the mutation
- Frataxin deficiency results in abnormal intramitochondrial iron accumulation, defective mitochondrial respiration, free radical overproduction, and oxidant-induced intracellular damage
- Cells of the nervous system, heart, and pancreas with high metabolic needs are particularly susceptible to free radical damage

Risk Factors

- Family history of Friedreich's ataxia

Clinical Features

- Slowly progressive lower limb ataxia starting at age 10 to 15 years
- Followed by dysarthria and upper limb ataxia
- Muscle weakness, lower limb spasticity, scoliosis, bladder dysfunction, absent lower limb reflexes, loss of position, and vibration sense
- 67% have hypertrophic cardiomyopathy with chest pain, shortness of breath, and heart palpitations
- 30% have diabetes mellitus

Natural History

- Average onset age of 10 to 15 years, with most before 25 years, with gait ataxia the first symptom (spinocerebellar degeneration leads to proprioception loss)
- Within 5 years of onset, patients develop "scanning" dysarthria, lower limb weakness, and decreased joint-position, and vibration sense distally. This is due to degeneration of the dorsal root ganglia, posterior columns, corticospinal tracts, dorsal spinocerebellar tracts, and the cerebellum.

Diagnosis

Differential diagnosis

- Amyotrophic lateral sclerosis
- B12 deficiency
- Syphilis
- Peripheral neuropathy
- Hereditary motor sensory neuropathies
- Spinal cord compression
- Ovarian cancer
- Mitochondrial disorders
- Ataxia with vitamin E deficiency
- Slow virus (Creutzfeldt-Jakob disease)
- Phenytoin intoxication

History

- Diagnostic criteria:
  - Disease duration >5 years
  - Disease onset age <25 years (96%)
  - Progressive ataxia of gait and limbs
  - Absent lower limb muscle stretch reflexes (88%)
  - Extensor plantar response

Examination

- General: kyphoscoliosis
- Head, eyes, ears, nose, and throat (HEENT): nystagmus
- Cardiac: murmurs
- Extremities: pes cavus (short foot, high arch, hammer toes), limb weakness, spasticity
- Neuro: ataxia of four limbs, cerebellar dysarthria, loss of vibratory and position sense, high steppage gait, positive Babinski reflex, absent lower limb reflexes

Testing

- Molecular genetic testing
- Targeted mutation analysis by polymerase chain reaction and/or Southern blot analysis of the GAA repeat

- EMG/nerve conduction study (NCS) with motor nerve conduction velocities >40 m/sec, with reduced or absent sensory nerve action potentials and absent H-reflex
- Electrocardiogram and echocardiogram for a baseline of cardiomyopathy
- Blood tests: fasting glucose, vitamin E, and B12 levels
- Magnetic resonance imaging (MRI) of the brain and spine to rule out other brain and spinal cord neurologic conditions

Pitfalls

- 25% of individuals homozygous for GAA expansion have atypical findings:
  - Late onset at age 26 to 39 years, at times >40 years
  - Retained reflexes
  - Spastic paraparesis without ataxia

Red flags

- Shortness of breath on exertion, dizziness, syncope, chest pain, or arrhythmias

Treatment

Medical

- Idebenone (analog of coenzyme Q10, free radical scavenger) 5 mg/kg improves left ventricular heart mass, no significant effect on ataxia
- Erythropoietin (frataxin expression upregulator)— ongoing research
- Medications for spasticity, arrhythmias, diabetes, bladder dysfunction
- Psychological support

Exercises

- Muscle-strengthening exercises not effective
- Physical therapy/occupational therapy (PT/OT) for spasticity, to maintain flexibility, and prevent contractures
- Speech therapy for dysphagia management

Modalities

- Bracing for pes cavus and kyphoscoliosis
- Prostheses: walking aids or wheelchairs for mobility

Injection

- Botulinum toxin for spasticity

Surgical

- Correct foot deformities and scoliosis
- Gastrostomy for dysphagia
- Pacemaker insertion

Consults

- Neurology
- Genetics
- Physical medicine and rehabilitation

Complications of treatment

- Medications for spasticity: includes sedation and central nervous system depression

Prognosis

- Larger GAA expansions are associated with earlier disease onset, increased frequency of cardiomyopathy and upper limb areflexia, and more rapid disease progression
- Most patients are wheelchair-bound 15 to 20 years after symptom onset
- Average age of death is 37 years, often due to cardiac failure and aspiration pneumonia
- Average interval from symptoms onset to death is 36 years in more recent studies

Helpful Hints

- First symptom is usually unsteady gait; later, ataxia gradually worsens, affecting the arms and then the trunk
- Genetic counseling of the family is important

Suggested Readings

Bidichandani SI, Delatycki MB. *Friedreich Ataxia.* GeneReviews; 1998 Dec 18 [updated 2009 Jun 25]. [Internet].

Pagon RA, Bird TD, Dolan CR, et al., eds. Seattle, WA: University of Washington, Seattle; 1993–2011.

www.ncbi.nlm.nih.gov/bookshelf/br.fcgi?book=gene&part =friedreich

Huntington's Disease

Gabriel Smith MD ■ Nathan D. Prahlow MD

Description

Huntington's disease (HD) is a progressive, fatal, autosomal dominant disorder characterized by motor, behavioral, and cognitive dysfunction.

Etiology/Types

- Autosomal dominant hereditary increase in polyglutamine (CAG) repeats in the gene coding sequence of the Huntingtin gene
- Westphal variant (~10% of HD cases)—onset at age <20 years, characterized by Parkinsonian features with little or no choreiform movements

Epidemiology

- Prevalence of two to eight cases per 100,000
- Onset is typically between 25 and 45 years (range of 3–70 years)
- Male-to-female ratio is 1:1

Pathogenesis

- Genetic disorder resulting in abnormal protein production and cell death in the basal ganglia
  - Genetic anticipation occurs resulting in increasing numbers of repeats with subsequent generations
- CAG repeats result in Huntingtin protein dysfunction
- Dysfunction of protein (unknown function) leads to disturbed homeostasis within neurons
- Neurodegeneration in the basal ganglia results in clinical features of HD

Risk Factors

- Positive family history
- Age 25 to 45 years

Clinical Features

- Progressive, involuntary choreiform movements
- Changes in behavior
- Changes in personality
- Dementia

Natural History

- Symptoms may begin at any age and are progressive
- Chorea: jerky, random, uncontrollable movements
- Difficulty with chewing, swallowing, speaking, and ambulating all progress over time
- Cognitive abilities decline progressively
- Full-time care is eventually required
- Life expectancy is approximately 20 years after the onset of symptoms

Diagnosis

Differential diagnosis

- Neuroacanthocytosis
- Multiple sclerosis
- Systemic lupus erythematosus
- HIV
- Cocaine or other central nervous system stimulants

History

- Gradually increasing, unintentional choreiform movement over months to years
- Dysarthria and dysphagia are common
- Personality changes
- Poor memory and intellectual dysfunction
- Depression, psychosis, and suicidal ideation are common

Examination

- Generalized choreiform movements, often disguised by the patient as purposeful actions
- Manifestations of mood disorder (variable)
- Dysphonia
- May appear parkinsonian in later disease

Testing

- Head computed tomography/magnetic resonance imaging (CT/MRI) looking for caudate atrophy
- Genetic testing for CAG repeats
- May consider genetically testing children
- HIV testing
- Antiphospholipid antibodies
- Urine drug screen

Pitfalls

- Delayed diagnosis
- Patients with HD often need 24-hour care as disease progresses

Red flags

- Loss of coordination, leading to frequent falls
- Suicidal ideation or behavior

Treatment

Medical
- Benzodiazepines
- Valproic acid
- Tetrabenazine—dopamine depleting agent
- Selective serotonin re-uptake inhibitors (SSRIs) for depression
- Atypical antipsychotics preferred for treatment of psychosis

Exercises
- Core strengthening for posture
- Coordination improvement
- Speech therapy to prevent aspiration

Modalities
- None

Surgical
- None

Consults
- Neurology
- Psychiatry, with individual, group, and family therapy sessions

- Genetic Counseling
- Physical therapy/occupational therapy (PT/OT)
- Speech therapy
- Physical medicine and rehabilitation

Complications of treatment
- Standard side-effect profiles of medications

Prognosis
- Progression of disease and death is inevitable
- Earlier age of onset in subsequent generations

Helpful Hints
- Clinical diagnosis of HD can be strongly suspected in cases of chorea with a positive family history
- Open communication with genetic counselors is vital if children of HD patients are considering being tested for the disease

Suggested Reading
Sturrock A, Leavitt B. The clinical and genetic features of Huntington disease. *J Geriatr Psychiatry Neurol.* 2010;23(4):243–259.

VII: Movement Disorders

Parkinson's Disease

Shangming Zhang MD FAAPMR

Description

Parkinson's disease (PD) is the most common movement disorder. It occurs as a result of degeneration of brain stem nuclei, especially the dopaminergic cells of substantia nigra. Hyperactivity of the cholinergic neurons in the caudate nuclei is also thought to contribute to PD. The common clinical features include resting tremor, rigidity, postural instability, and bradykinesia.

Etiology/Types

- Due to lack of dopamine-producing cells in the basal ganglia

Epidemiology

- Prevalence: 160 per 100,000
- 1% of the population over 50 years of age

Pathogenesis

- Dopamine depletion leads to imbalance between dopaminergic input and cholinergic input

Risk Factors

- Age: 5 per 100,000 in the population younger than 40 years *versus* 300 to 700 per 100,000 in the population at 70 years of age
- Male-to-female ratio of 3:2

Clinical Features

- Resting tremor (the most common presentation)
- Lead pipe rigidity (constant increase in tone resisting movement)
- Cogwheel rigidity (jerky increases in tone resisting movement)
- Postural instability
- Bradykinesia

Natural History

- Chronic progressive debilitating neurodegenerative central nervous system disease

Diagnosis

Differential diagnosis

- Drug-induced parkinsonism
- Toxin-induced parkinsonism
- Multiple strokes
- Wilson's disease
- Normal pressure hydrocephalus
- Brain tumors

History

- Resting "pill-rolling" tremor suppressed by activity or sleep
- Smooth resistance to passive movement and joint range of motion
- Festinating gait, with small, shuffling steps
- Frequent falls or tripping
- Masked facies
- Small handwriting (micrographia)
- Depression
- Dementia

Examination

- Mask-like facies
- Muscle rigidity
- Resting tremor
- General slowing of movements
- Postural instability
- Olfactory dysfunction
- Micrographia

Testing

- Plasma ceruloplasmin and copper to rule out Wilson's disease
- Brain magnetic resonance imaging (MRI) to rule out normal pressure hydrocephalus, tumor, multiple strokes, subdural hematoma

Pitfalls

- Driving evaluation
- Fall prevention: home evaluation
- Aspiration pneumonia: swallowing evaluation

Red flags

- Orthostatic hypotension
- Aspiration pneumonia

Treatment

Medical

- L-dopa: levodopa/carbidopa
- Dopamine receptor agonists: pergolide, bromocriptine
- Anticholinergics: amantadine, benztropine
- Dopamine metabolism inhibitors: selegiline

Exercise

- Physical exercises improve physical functioning, health-related quality of life, strength, balance, and gait for patients with PD
- Treadmill training beneficial

Modalities

- Deep brain stimulator effectively reduces tremor, rigidity, and bradykinesia
- Biofeedback for sialorrhea

Injections

- Chemodenervation with botulinum toxin to treat spasticity and tremor

Surgical

- Destructive surgeries: thalamotomy and pallidotomy
- Deep brain stimulation
- To be used to treat rigidity, dyskinesia, and tremor in advanced PD patients who are unresponsive to or intolerant of oral medications

Consults

- Neurology for medication options
- Physical and occupational therapy
- Speech language pathology
- Psychiatry for management of depression and dementia
- Neurosurgery for surgical treatment in advanced cases

Complications of treatment

- Side effects of medications
- Infection or failure of surgery

Prognosis

- Positive prognostic indicators: early tremor, rigidity, and a family history of Parkinson's disease
- Negative prognostic indicators: bradykinesia, akinesia, postural instability, gait dysfunction, cognitive deficits, dysphagia, and late age of onset
- Mortality rate from PD is threefold that of the general population matched for age, gender, and race

Helpful Hint

- L-dopa is currently a keystone of treatment and has shown to reduce mortality by 50%

Suggested Reading

Doherty J, Fried G, Saulino M. Degenerative movement disorders of the central nervous system. In: Braddom RL, ed. *Physical Medicine & Rehabilitation*. 4th ed. (pp. 1223–1232). Philadelphia, PA: Elsevier Saunders; 2011.

Torticollis

Shashank J. Davé DO FAAPMR

Description

Abnormal head/neck muscle contraction resulting in aberrant movement or posture of the head, neck, or shoulders

Etiology/Types

- Sagittal plane: *anterocollis*–forward flexion
- Sagittal plane: *retrocollis*–backward extension
- Coronal plane: *laterocollis*–sidebending
- Transverse plane: *torticollis*–rotation
- Usually involves combinations of the above

Epidemiology

- Focal dystonia: cervical dystonia is the most common type
- Prevalence of focal dystonia 295 per million
- Incidence of focal dystonia 24 per million

Pathogenesis

- Lesions within the basal ganglia, motor cortex, and cerebellum
- Neurotransmitter imbalance in dopamine and acetylcholine

Risk Factors

- Neck injury (eg, motor vehicle collision)
- Stressful life events

Clinical Features

- Head/neck muscle spasm with involuntary sustained tonic or clonic contractions
- Co-contraction: simultaneous agonist and antagonist contraction
- Contractions may intensify with voluntary effort
- Sensory trick: light touch over affected body region (eg, chin) may attenuate dystonia

Natural History

- Average onset age 30 to 50 years
- Usually waxes and wanes, but may spontaneously remit
- May progress to other body regions, such as the face

Diagnosis

Differential diagnosis

- Cervical radiculopathy
- Myofascial pain syndrome
- Cervical myelopathy
- Soft tissue strain
- Stroke
- Brain injury
- Medication side effects (dopamine antagonists)
- Multiple sclerosis

History

- Neck pain (50%)
- Functionally limiting neck range of motion
- Head/neck tremor
- May worsen with stress

Examination

- Extremities:
  - May have associated tremor/dystonia if progression
  - Usually normal strength and reflexes
- Neurologic:
  - Neck muscle tenderness
  - Asymmetric head/neck position and/or range of motion in sagittal, coronal, or transverse plane, or combination of all the three
  - Associated trigger points

Testing

- Cervical spine x-ray and magnetic resonance imaging (MRI) to rule out other causes and structural abnormalities
- Needle EMG to determine which muscles are involved in torsion pattern
- Brain MRI to rule out other conditions

Pitfalls

- Missing myofascial pain syndrome

Red flags

- Cervical cord compression
- Malignancy

Treatment

Medical

- Muscle relaxants: baclofen, tizanidine
- Analgesics

Exercises

- Isotonic neck strengthening
- Muscle energy/proprioceptive neuromuscular facilitation
- Multiplanar range of motion

Modalities
- EMG biofeedback
- Heat/ultrasound
- Ice

Injection
- Botulinum toxin

Surgical
- Deep brain stimulation

Consults
- Neurology
- Physical medicine and rehabilitation
- Neurosurgery

Complications of treatment
- Oral muscle relaxants: drowsiness and dizziness
- Botulinum toxin: neck muscle weakness, dysphagia, xerostomia

Prognosis
- May very rarely spontaneously remit, but cervical dystonia is considered a lifelong neurodegenerative disorder

Helpful Hints
- On examination, break down torsion pattern into three cardinal planes to determine which muscles may be involved (transverse plane/toricollis may involve contralateral sternocleidomastoid and ipsilateral splenius capitis)
- Needle localization techniques with botulinum toxin injections include EMG and ultrasound

Suggested Readings
Comella CL. The treatment of cervical dystonia with botulinum toxins. *J Neural Transm.* 2008;115(4):579–583. [Epub 2007 Nov 12].

Stacy M. Role of botulinum toxin in the treatment of cervical dystonia. *Neurol Clin.* 2008;26(Suppl 1):23.

Tourette's Syndrome

Susan X. Yu DO ■ Shashank J. Davé DO FAAPMR

Description

A chronic childhood-onset condition characterized by motor and vocal tics lasting for more than 1 year. Motor tics include simple (twitching, eye blinking), dystonic (slow twisting movements), tonic (isometric contractions), complex motor (touching, tapping), and echopraxia (mimicking gestures of others). Vocal/phonic tics include simple (throat clearing, sniffing, coughing), complex (words or partial words), coprolalia (shouted obscenities), and echolalia (repeating words of others)

Etiology/Types

- Primary: unknown
- Secondary:
  - Inherited: majority of cases, but no gene identified
  - Infection: *Streptococcus* infection (not yet proven)
  - Toxins: hypothesized
  - Traumatic brain injury

Epidemiology

- 1% prevalence
- Rare in African descent

Pathogenesis

- Unclear. May be due to a developmental defect in the migration of the GABAergic neurons in the basal ganglia creating an imbalance in the cortico-striato-thalamic circuit. Tics are hypothesized to be a result of failure of cortical inhibition of unwanted motor programs that are generated in the basal ganglia
- Postulated autoimmune reaction after streptococcal infection; however, no temporal link has been found

Risk Factors

- Comorbid Obsessive-Compulsive Disorder (OCD)
- Maternal prenatal use of coffee, cigarettes, and alcohol
- Nonspecific maternal life stress during pregnancy
- Forceps delivery
- Low birth weight
- Likely bilineal (maternal and paternal) transmission

Clinical Features

- Involuntary, sudden, rapid, brief, repetitive head, neck movements, gestures and vocalizations during times of stress, anxiety, excitement, fatigue, or boredom
- Boys are more likely to have tics with attention deficit hyperactivity disorder (ADHD)
- Girls are more likely to have tics with OCD

Natural History

- Average onset age 5.6 years
- Tics most severe at age 10 years
- Tics start to resolve at age 13 years
- One-third resolve in adulthood
- Tics may not resolve until age 30 years

Diagnosis

Differential diagnosis

- A diagnosis of Tourette's syndrome includes each of the following:
  - Onset younger than 18 years
  - Both a motor tic and a phonic tic present for over 1 year
  - Tics occurring many times a day—usually in bouts—and nearly every day; however, some may be present only intermittently
  - Not due to the direct physiological effects of a substance (stimulants) or general medical condition (Huntington's disease or postviral encephalitis)
- Allergies
- Asthma
- Hyperactivity, nervousness
- Dystonia
- Myoclonus
- Chorea
- Compulsions

History

- Tics decreased by sleep, alcohol, orgasm, fever, relaxation and concentrating on an enjoyable task
- Suppression of tic in public places, until an irresistible impulse to release the tic
- Waxing and waning of tics
- Premonitory sensation localized at the site of the tic

Examination

- Except for tics, neurologic exam is usually normal

Testing

- Clinical diagnosis
- Neuroimaging and laboratory tests not needed

- Magnetic resonance imaging (MRI) shows overall larger amygdala and hippocampus volume (but decreases with age)
- Electroencephalography and evoked responses not helpful

Pitfalls
- Assess for coexisting psychiatric conditions, especially ADHD and OCD
- Need to rule out benign common tic disorder that lasts <1 year in 3% to 24% of school children
- Vocal tics may be due to upper respiratory disorders

Red flags
- Seizures
- Fever/infection
- Head trauma

Treatment

Medical
- Education about the condition is key in order to maintain and strengthen the child's self-confidence and self-esteem
- Habit-reversal treatment to suppress tics
- Commonly used medications may or may not be Food and Drug Administration approved for treatment of Tourette's syndrome
- Tics alone:
  - First line: guanfacine, tetrabenazine
  - Second line: fluphenazine, risperidone, atypical antipsychotics (haloperidol, pimozide), clonzaepam, topriamate, botulinum toxin
  - Third line: deep brain stimulation
- With OCD:
  - First line: cognitive behavioral therapy, selective serotonin re-uptake inhibitors (SSRIs)
  - Second line: atypical antipsychotics (haloperidol, pimozide)
  - Third line: deep brain stimulation
- With ADHD:
  - First line: behavioral therapy, guanfacine
  - Second line: clonidine, methylphenidate, other central nervous system stimulants, atomoxetine

Exercises
- None

Modalities
- None

Injection
- Botulinum toxin for eye blinking, neck and shoulder tics

Surgical
- Deep brain stimulation of the thalamus, globus pallidus, putamen, subthalamic nucleus

Consults
- Neurology
- Allergy
- Ophthalmology

Complications of treatment
- Atypical antipsychotics: marked weight gain, glucose intolerance
- All antipsychotics: sedation, depression, increased appetite, parkinsonism

Prognosis
- In one-third of children, tics resolve in adulthood
- In one-third of children, tics become much less severe
- In one-third of children, there is no change in tics
- Tic severity stabilizes by age 25 years

Helpful Hints
- Best time to look for tics is when the patient is walking into or out of the exam room
- Tetrabenazine causes less weight gain and less tardive dyskinesia than antipsychotic medications
- Methylphenidate is effective for ADHD and does not exacerbate tics

Suggested Readings
Jankovic J, Kurlan R. Tourette syndrome: Evolving concepts. *Mov Disord.* 2011;26(6):1149–56, May.

Kurlan R. Clinical practice. Tourette's syndrome. *N Engl J Med.* 2010;363(24):2332–2338. (Review). (Erratum in: *N Engl J Med.* 2011 Feb 3;364(5):490).

VII: Movement Disorders

Writer's Cramp

Susan X. Yu DO ■ Nathan D. Prahlow MD

Description

A focal task-specific dystonia, an involuntary spasm, flexion, extension, and or rotation of fingers, wrist, elbow and or shoulder, causing writing difficulties

Etiology/Types

- Etiology unknown, autosomal dominant gene with incomplete penetrance
- Simple: writing difficulty without difficulty performing other manual motor tasks
- Progressive: writing difficulty along with difficulty with other motor tasks such as hair combing and lifting utensils
- Dystonic: involuntary hand spasm that interferes with many manual motor functions

Epidemiology

- 69 per million
- Most common in the age group 30 to 50 years
- Male-to-female ratio is 1.3:1
- Occupations that involve writing

Pathogenesis

- Unknown
- Likely a disorder of a motor subroutine in the cortex-basal ganglia-thalamus-cortex loop
- Spinal reciprocal inhibition, a process that inhibits the antagonist muscles when the agonist muscles are active, is reduced
- Multichannel EMG of the affected side shows excessive simultaneous contraction of agonist and antagonist active hand muscles when writing, with abnormally prolonged EMG activation bursts, especially in the triceps

Risk Factors

- 5% with positive family history
- 25% with relatives with dystonia
- Higher risk with history of local trauma

Clinical Features

- Excessive co-contraction of agonist and antagonist active hand muscles when writing (normal: alternating contraction of agonist and antagonist muscles when writing)

Natural History

- Some patients progress from simple to dystonic writer's cramp

Diagnosis

Differential diagnosis

- Benign essential tremor
- Parkinson's disease
- Multiple sclerosis
- Spinocerebellar degeneration
- Spinal muscular atrophy
- Dopamine-responsive dystonia
- Wilson's disease

History

- Progressive writing difficulty
- Pain is rare, but may have finger, forearm, arm, or shoulder discomfort

Examination

- Flexion and wrist ulnar deviation, elbow elevation when writing
- Compensatory maneuvers: excessive gripping; or holding pen vertically, in a closed fist, or between index and long fingers
- Normal muscle strength, muscle stretch reflexes, and sensation
- Decreased range of motion and increased muscle tone in the flexor and extensor muscles of the upper limb
- One-third of patients with large-amplitude hand tremor during writing or when arm is outstretched

Testing

- EMG of both extremities to rule out nerve injury
- Magnetic resonance imaging (MRI) of the brain to rule out a structural lesion

Pitfalls

- A small number of patients may have pain and paresthesias due to carpal tunnel syndrome, caused by repeated dystonic wrist spasms

Red flags

- A focal dystonia can sometimes be the first manifestation of a generalized dystonia

Treatment

Medical

- Anticholinergic: Trihexyphenidyl, effective in 5%:
  - Reduces dystonia by blocking cholinergic innervation of the basal ganglia, which in turn increases the dopaminergic output
- Beta-adrenergic blockers: propranolol:
  - Reduce hand tremor

Exercises

- None

Modalities

- Occupational therapy—adaptive devices:
  - Alter pen grip, increase pen diameter, use a writing devise that mounts a pen on a gliding or ball-bearing tripod frame (Blackburn writing devise)
- Sensory discrimination therapy
- Transcutaneous electrical nerve stimulation (TENS) of forearm flexors improves writing time and decrease tremor
- Cooling and warming of arm with various modalities may allow better writing performance

Injection

- Botulinum toxin with EMG guidance to weaken overactive muscles: effective in 67%

Surgical

- Stereotactic thalamotomy
- Deep brain stimulation of the ventral thalamic nucleus (Voa and Vop: nucleus ventrooralis anterior and posterior)

Consults

- Neurology
- Neurosurgery
- Physical medicine and rehabilitation

Complications of treatment

- Trihexyphenidyl: dry mouth, blurred vision, memory loss, confusion
- Botulinum toxin: temporary weakness and pain at injection sites

Prognosis

- 33% attempt to change hands for writing
- 50% continue to use dominant hand for writing
- 20% to 25% develop same symptoms on the contralateral hand and forearm
- 15% discontinue writing with dominant hand
- 5% have spontaneous remission for months or years, but with eventual recurrence
- 7% develop carpal tunnel syndrome

Helpful Hint

- Writer's cramp is more likely to cause coordination deficits rather than to cause pain, as in overuse syndromes

Suggested Readings

Gordon NS. Focal dystonia, with special reference to writer's cramp. *Int J Clin Pract.* 2005;59(9):1088–1090.

Rhoad RC, Stern PJ. Writer's cramp—a focal dystonia: Etiology, diagnosis, and treatment. *J Hand Surg Am.* 1993;18(3): 541–544.